Pregnant Drug Addict

Edited by

Catherine Siney

SRN, RM

Chapters by:
Peter Carey
Lyn Matthews
Merseyside Drugs Council
Clive Morrison
Sue Ruben
Colette Sparey and Steve Walkinshaw

Books for Midwives Press

Books for Midwives Press is a joint collaboration
between The Royal College of Midwives and
Haigh & Hochland Publications Ltd.

Published by Books for Midwives Press, 174a Ashley Road, Hale, Cheshire, WA15 9SF, England

© 1995, Catherine Siney
First edition

ISBN1-898507-13-9

British Library Cataloguing in Publication Data
A catalogue record for this book is available from the British Library

Printed in Great Britain by Cromwell Press Ltd

Contents

Introduction: CATHERINE SINEY   *v*

Chapter One: CATHERINE SINEY
Management of Pregnant Women who are Drug-dependent   1

Chapter Two: SUE RUBEN
Women and Drug Use   9

Chapter Three: CLIVE L MORRISON
Medical Problems of Illicit Drug Misuse in Pregnancy and
Harm Minimization   15

Chapter Four: COLETTE SPAREY AND STEVE WALKINSHAW
Obstetric Problems for Drug Users   24

Chapter Five: PETER CAREY
Hepatitis B, Pregnancy and the Drug User   34

Chapter Six: PETER CAREY
HIV, Pregnancy and the Drug User   42

Chapter Seven: CLIVE L MORRISON
The Sexual Health Needs of Female Drug Users   51

Chapter Eight: PETER CAREY
Sexually Transmitted Diseases, Pregnancy and the Drug User   58

Chapter Nine: LYN MATTHEWS
Outreach Work with Female Sex Workers in Liverpool   83

Chapter Ten: MERSEYSIDE DRUGS COUNCIL
Drugs Counselling and the Pregnant Addict   92

Conclusion: CATHERINE SINEY   99

References and Bibliography   100

Appendices
I: Liverpool Neonatal Drug Withdrawal Chart   110
II: Poster   112
III: Information about the Care of Pregnant Substance Abusers   113

Acknowledgements

I would like to thank the staff of the Liverpool Women's Hospital, the staff of the Liverpool and Sefton Drug Agencies – both statutory and non-statutory, and all the community staff who have helped and supported me since the service begain in Liverpool in March 1990.

A special thank you to my husband for his moral and clerical support.

Introduction

CATHERINE SINEY

This book has been put together to give an introduction to health care professionals on the subject of opiate-dependent women and pregnancy. Although many drugs are abused, at the present time the main drug of abuse remains heroin. Between 60 and 80 known drug-dependent women are delivered annually in the Liverpool Women's Hospital (formerly Liverpool Maternity Hospital, Mill Road Maternity Hospital and The Women's Hospital) and a specialist service for these women has been available since 1990. In 1990 I looked around for a book which would give me an overview of the subject and could not find one. I wanted to know about the history of drug abuse, where the systems for drug treatment programmes came from and the effects of drugs on the fetus and neonate as well as the woman. I hope that this book will at least go part of the way to explaining these and other points. The people I asked to contribute a chapter all have extensive experience in their field and I felt that it would be good to have the benefit of their experience to give a broad picture of this extremely complex subject. Some of the chapters will overlap but this will allow them to be read on their own.

Historical background

In the 19th century opiate use was widespread in Britain, as well as North America and parts of Europe. Opium and laudanum were used by the middle classes for self-medication, the literary and bohemian circles indulged for experimentation and the working classes used them as intoxicants and aids to physical labour. During the course of the industrial revolution there were public health concerns about workers' use of opiates and also the practice of 'infant doping' with remedies such as 'Soothing Syrup' and 'Mothers' Quietness'. In the late 19th century there were vivid accounts of opium dens in the East End of London which led to further concerns and anxieties about the moral welfare of the working classes.

In the 18th and early 19th centuries the approach became more medically orientated. The Pharmacy Act 1868 restricted the sales of morphine and opium by pharmacists and prohibited their sale by grocers and general stores; in 1908 the Poisons and Pharmacy Act regulated the sale of patent medicines. Medical practitioners made various attempts to extend the provisions of the Inebriates Act in 1888 to cover those who became dependent on opiates, but lost. The Inebriates Act allowed for voluntary detention of 'habitual drunkards' and 'inebriates'. However the Lunacy Act of 1890 was sometimes applied to drug addicts. This act allowed for a form of guardianship for patients deemed incapable of managing their affairs and property. In 1913 the Mental Deficiency Act was specific legislation by which any sedative, narcotic or stimulant drug fell within the definition of an 'intoxicant'; this then allowed for people who were deemed 'moral imbeciles' to be confined within an institution or placed under guardianship. British opinion was divided in 1914; addiction was seen as either a medical problem to be treated or a vice to be controlled through penal sanctions. During World War I (1914–1918) there was great concern about the spread of cocaine and a regulation was introduced under the Defence of the Realms Act (DORA 40B) which prohibited the possession of cocaine unless supplied on prescription. The Dangerous Drugs Acts of 1920 and 1923 made possession of opiates and cocaine illegal unless supplied by a doctor and the Home Secretary was authorized to regulate manufacture, distribution and sale of these substances. These Acts brought addiction into the criminal model of action but the Rolleston Committee (Departmental Committee on Morphine and Heroin Addiction) was established in 1924 by the Ministry of Health,

> 'to consider and advise on the circumstances, if any, in which the supply of morphine and heroin ... to persons suffering from addiction to those drugs may be regarded as medically advisable and as to the precautions which it is advisable that medical practitioners administering or prescribing morphine or heroin should adopt for the avoidance of abuse'.

The recommendations of the committee were that the prescription of heroin and morphine to certain classes of addicts was to be deemed a 'legitimate medical treatment' and that control of prescribing practices was to be by professional self-regulation through a medical panel. However, unauthorized possession of certain substances remained a criminal offence.

The Interdepartmental Committee on Drug Addiction was convened in 1958 to review existing policy and concluded that addiction to dangerous drugs was still a small problem. It was reconvened in 1962 and in 1964 there was great public concern about amphetamines ('pep pills' and 'purple hearts') and cannabis use among young people. Also the number of known heroin addicts had risen from 47 to 328 over a five-year period (1959–1964) and the total number of known addicts rose from 260 in 1954 to 753 in 1964. They recommended tighter controls on the supply of drugs to addicts, these controls to take the form of a system of notification, to a central authority, by doctors of any unregistered addicts with whom they came into professional contact. Specialist drug treatment centres were to be established, at least in the London area, with only the staff there retaining the right to prescribe heroin and cocaine to drug addicts, and these treatment centres should have powers to detain addicts for compulsory treatment if this was felt to be necessary. All except the recommendation to detain for compulsory treatment were put into the Dangerous Drugs Act of 1967, and subsequently in April of 1968 regulations were introduced that prohibited ordinary medical practitioners from prescribing heroin and cocaine to addicts.

In the 1970s the clinics transferred patients from heroin (which was injected) onto injectable methadone as a substitute and then moved towards prescription of oral methadone as treatment in either detoxification or maintenance regimes. In 1983 there was a 42 per cent increase in the number of addicts notified to the Home Office, almost entirely confined to heroin misuse. In 1984 there were 5,190 addicts receiving methadone in the United Kingdom, but by 1987 this number had increased to 9,763. Methadone was the first completely synthetic opiate-light drug. It was developed in Germany during World War II and appeared in the United States in the late 1940s.

The heroin epidemic which emerged in the 1980s was associated with the arrival of heroin which was cheap and plentiful; this came from Southwest Asia. Heroin misuse became a serious problem in many towns and cities in the north of England and Scotland where heroin had been largely unknown. Research papers began to be published detailing a sharp increase in places like Glasgow and Edinburgh; also in Liverpool, Sheffield, Carlisle and Manchester. The scale was enormous; for example, in the Wirral peninsula (Cheshire) alone in 1987 detailed prevalence estimates indicated that there were some 5,000 regular heroin users when there had been fewer than a hundred people known to be using opiates in 1980. In one town in the Wirral peninsula, where the problem was particularly severe, as many as 8.6 per cent of 16–24 year olds were known heroin users (Parker et al, 1986). There was a tendency for heroin misuse to be associated with high levels of unemployment and other forms of social deprivation (Pearson, 1987).

This experience in the 1980s confirmed the tendency in America in an earlier period for heroin misuse to be associated with areas of urban deprivation. The realization that the Southwest Asian imported 'brown' heroin could be 'smoked' (the practice of 'chasing the dragon') helped to accelerate the growth of the heroin habit among people for whom self-injection would have proved a barrier. In areas such as Merseyside and Manchester, 'chasing the dragon' became the dominant route of administration.

In 1984 a ministerial sub-committee was appointed by the government who were alarmed at the increase in heroin misuse. The following year a strategy document was issued called *Tackling Drug Misuse*. Action on five main fronts was proposed:

a) reducing supplies from abroad;
b) making enforcement even more effective;
c) maintaining effective deterrents and tighter domestic controls;
d) developing prevention; and,
e) improving treatment and rehabilitation.

The two broad initiatives on the domestic front were the enhancement of health education programmes and a Central Funding Initiative (CFI) to improve services for drug misusers. The CFI led to the development of community-based services which have played a crucial role in limiting the spread of human immunodeficiency virus (HIV). These services at local level, which contain a range of advice and treatment options, remain a key part of overall HIV and drug misuse prevention. By 1990 there were 135 advice and counselling agencies, 75 community drug teams, 49 residential rehabilitation units, 33 drug dependency units and 200 needle exchange schemes.

Statistics

In March 1994 the Department of Health issued the first bulletin in a series containing aggregate information on those drug misusers attending services for problem drug misusers in England. Each bulletin covers a six-month period and includes new attenders rather than people already in contact with such services. The information, which reaches the Department of Health via the Regional Health Authority Drug Misuse Databases, includes the age group and sex of the person, the types of drugs misused, whether the drug is injected or not and the type of agency contacted.

The first bulletin gave information for the six months ending 31 March 1993 and found that 75 per cent of the 17,822 individuals attending services for problem drug misusers were male and 25 per cent were female. Ninety six per cent were aged between 15 and 44 years and 12 per cent were aged under 20 years. Heroin use accounted for 47 per cent of the total, with methadone (the heroin substitute) notified by treatment agencies who prescribe it to people in treatment, accounting for 15 per cent and the amphetamine group of drugs accounting for 11 per cent. In 38 per cent of cases the main drug used was injected. These bulletins will be in addition to the Home Office Addicts Index.

In 1992 the number of opiate or cocaine misusers notified nationally was 430 notifications per million population; the rate for the Mersey region was 1,537 per million population. Over 40 per cent of heroin, amphetamine and cocaine users in the Mersey region were reported to inject the drug. At the end of December 1992 the ratio of notified injecting addicts to injecting addicts who were HIV positive was 66.5:1 in the Mersey region compared to 2:1 in the Northern region and 2.4:1 in the North West Thames Region (due in the main to the early start of harm minimization policies). The total number of new drug addicts notified in the year 1992 to the Home Office by Regional Health Authorities for the United Kingdom was 9663. There were 1698 aged under 21 years, the average age overall for men was 27.1 years, the average age for women was 26.5 years. During 1992 15,040 addicts were renotified to the Home Office, the average age for men was 31.1 years and for women was 30 years. In 1991, 344 deaths of drug addicts were notified to the Home Office.

In 1993 a survey was undertaken to determine the prevalence of drug misuse in pregnancy and describe the services provided by maternity services for drug misusers (Morrison and Siney, 1995). A postal questionnaire was sent to 213 maternity units in England and Wales which asked about the extent of involvement with pregnant drug misusers, the services offered, the availability of liaison with drug treatment agencies and the policies on health care for neonates. The response rate was 89.3 per cent (191). There was an estimated number of 568 deliveries to drug misusers in a 12 month period. Only 29 per cent (57) of maternity units had formal links with local drug agencies and 52 per cent (100) automatically convened social service child care discussions. Fifty seven per cent (109) routinely admitted babies of drug misusing mothers to special care baby units and, although Hepatitis B screening was offered to women in 73 per cent (146) of the units, only 68 per cent (129) offered Hepatitis B prophlaxis to babies of women found infected in pregnancy. The results of the survey showed that local health purchasers should undertake needs assessment to ensure that discriminatory practices are not deterring women from seeking help.

The importance of effective antenatal care

The World Health Organisation (WHO) review of antenatal care (Rooney, 1992) stressed the importance of effective antenatal care in the future health and well-being of mothers and children. Education about pregnancy and childbirth should be started at an early age. The importance of good general health and planned pregnancy cannot be too heavily emphasized. Alcohol and tobacco in pregnancy are known to be detrimental to the health of the mother and the developing fetus and are associated with premature birth and low birthweight (Kline et al, 1987). Misuse of other drugs, for example opiates, is also associated with low birthweight and premature birth (Siney et al, 1995). Encouraging women who are dependent on drugs to let the maternity services know is very important. Identifying themselves gives them the chance to ask questions and allows professionals to give them choices. It empowers them, it gives them a chance to take control of an aspect of their life. Midwives must strive to find patterns of care that suit all women, not just the educationally and financially advantaged section of society. Care should be holistic, that is, it must look to not only the physical but also the social and financial needs.

While pregnancy will be a time of happiness, for many women, particularly those having their first child, it can be a time of great anxiety. They may worry about how parenthood and the responsibilities it brings will change their lives. Financial or housing problems may add to these anxieties. For the woman who is dependent on drugs all these anxieties are added to her addiction and, where illegal drugs are involved, the risky lifestyle that goes with it. Drug-taking women, especially those using opiates, may have reduced fertility and irregular or absent periods (Institute for the Study of Drug Dependency, 1992); it could therefore also be a huge shock for them to find themselves pregnant and the combination of shock and anxiety may make it difficult for some women to give up drugs and change their lifestyle. Many feel guilt about using drugs when pregnant but still are unable to give up their addiction. They may also fear, even when unjustified, that the unborn child or their existing children will be taken away if health or social workers find out about their drug use and may also fear being stigmatized when they go into hospital. It is vitally important that women who are drug-dependent are looked upon by maternity service personnel as pregnant women who misuse drugs rather than drug misusing women who are pregnant. If women are leading an illegal lifestyle then they may have lied to almost everyone they have come into contact with and that is why continuity of personnel is essential – this allows a relationship to develop and helps to engender an atmosphere of trust.

Another essential is that maternity service personnel should be aware of their attitudes towards pregnant drug misusers and should ensure that negative attitudes do not spoil the chance of a good relationship. If women are discouraged from attending antenatal care by the treatment they receive neither they nor their babies will receive the care they need, and studies in the United States from 1969–74 showed that illness in babies born to drug-dependent women was directly related to the amount of antenatal care they received (Connaughton and Reeser, 1977). Questioning for all women in the antenatal period should not simply be about the mother's general health and any drugs used, including tobacco and alcohol; the opportunity should also be used to educate about the risks to the fetus of all drugs taken during pregnancy. In this way drug use in the woman is seen as being an obstetric/paediatric concern, rather than a moral one.

Identification of women who are drug-dependent is not only of benefit to the mother and fetus, but also to the staff. Women who are cared for by staff who are not visibly disapproving of them or their lifestyle will find that problems expected when women are in-patients often do not materialize. Another important plus is that any social service concerns may be answered before the women are admitted to hospital and any decisions needed can be made before birth.

Confidentiality

The elaboration of the confidentiality clause 9 in the Code of Professional Conduct drawn up by the United Kingdom Central Council for Nursing, Midwifery and Health Visiting (UKCC) in 1987 says that information obtained in the course of professional practice shall be respected and that such information cannot be disclosed without the consent of the patient/client, or a person entitled to act on his or her behalf, except where disclosure is required by law or by the order of a court or is necessary to the public interest. A breach of confidentiality occurs if anyone deliberately or by accident gives information, which has been obtained in the course of professional practice, to a third party without the consent of the patient/client. The 'public interest', in the context of the UKCC advisory paper on confidentiality (UKCC, 1987), is taken to mean the interest of an individual, of groups of individuals or society as a whole and would encompass matters such as serious crime, child abuse and drug trafficking. (*Trafficking* – 'to deal or bargain in something that should not be the subject of trade'. The Concise Oxford Dictionary of Current English.)

There is no statutory right to confidentiality but there is also nothing to stop an aggrieved individual bringing a common law case before a civil court alleging breach of confidentiality and seeking financial recompense. Information shared with other professionals in the health and social work fields is shared in the belief that this is in the interest of the patient/client. Legislation covering data protection and its associated codes is not intended to prevent the exchange of information between professional staff who share the care of the patient/client. It is the duty of the practitioner to ensure as far as is possible that information shared is in strict professional confidence and for a specific purpose and in all cases she or he must be able to justify the decision. It may be appropriate for a practitioner to consult with their professional organization.

Legal 'requirements'

Contrary to what some health care professionals may believe, it is possible to be a parent and a drug misuser. The second report on drug-using parents and their children produced by the Standing Conference on Drug Abuse (SCODA, 1989), along with another report by the Social Services Inspectorate (1991), make it clear that drug misuse in itself is not sufficient reason to separate mother and child. The Children Act 1989 contains many principles and provisions, but an overriding principle is that in all court proceedings the welfare of the child will be paramount. In deciding what happens to a child the court has to consider the wishes of the child (in the light of age and understanding). If a local authority wishes to separate a parent from a child they have to show that the child's interest will be better served with separation and they have to demonstrate that the child would come to significant harm if left in his or her environment, and that the harm is attributable to the care being given to the child.

'Significant harm' is defined thus, 'where the question of whether harm suffered by the child is significant turns on the child's health or development, [this] shall be compared with that which could be reasonably expected of a similar child' (Institute for the Study of Drug Dependency, 1992).

Effects of drugs on pregnancy and the neonate

It is generally accepted that drugs should be prescribed in pregnancy only if the benefit to the mother is thought to be greater than the risk to the fetus. During the first trimester they may produce congenital malformations, that is they may be teratogenic, and during the second and third trimesters they may affect growth and functional development. Women who misuse drugs may not be in contact with any agency who is able to tell them about possible risks to their baby if they take drugs, including tobacco and alcohol, during pregnancy, but it is also important to remember that many of the obstetric problems commonly associated with illicit drug use are also associated with social deprivation and poor health and nutrition. However in Liverpool we found that things were not necessarily so bad as they seemed. The results of a retrospective case-control study comparing the outcomes of pregnancy of 103 opiate-dependent women who were on a methadone programme, and who received regular antenatal care, with women who were matched by age, parity and postal code who were not known to be drug misusers, showed that apart from an increased risk of prematurity and a reduction in birthweight the outcomes were broadly similar (Siney et al, 1995).

More specific effects of drugs on pregnancy are discussed in the chapter 'Obstetric care for drug users'. Intravenous injection of drugs runs the risk of both local and systemic infection (see chapters on medical problems, HIV and Hepatitis B).

It is important to remember that there is a difference between drug misuse and drug dependence. Drug misuse, which is broadly equivalent to 'drug abuse' and 'problem drug taking', denotes drug taking which is hazardous or harmful and unsanctioned by professional or cultural standards. Drug dependence is a term used to describe the altered physical and psychological state which results in disturbed physical and mental functioning when the drug is abruptly discontinued. It is broadly equivalent to 'drug addiction'. However not all drug misusers are drug-dependent (HMSO, 1991). Generally drugs on which women are dependent are likely to cause problems for the baby when it is withdrawn from the source, that is after birth. Symptoms of withdrawal vary in strength and effect dependent probably on the condition of the baby after birth. This would explain the wide variation in symptoms seen even when women have taken broadly similar amounts of illicit drugs. Mild symptoms may include sneezing, yawning, poor feeding, tremors when disturbed and loose stools; severe symptoms may include convulsions, tremors when undisturbed, nonstop high-pitched cry, sleeping less than an hour after a good feed and watery stools and projectile vomiting. Mild symptoms, when the baby can be comforted and continues to feed, will not probably require treatment, but treatment will be necessary if the baby becomes dehydrated, has convulsions or its agitation cannot be comforted. Treatment should make the baby comfortable enough to take a feed and settle down afterwards. The aim should be to wean the baby away from dependence and enable him or her to feed normally.

In 1985 Strang and Moran of the Manchester Regional Drug Dependence Unit recommended that opiate withdrawal symptoms should be treated by giving an opiate and then weaning down but not sedating the child; if the maternal addiction is to barbiturates then the baby should be weaned off with phenobarbitone and if the maternal addiction is to benzodiazepines then the baby should be treated with diazepam. In Liverpool we have been treating severe opiate withdrawal symptoms in the neonate by giving morphine sulphate orally and reducing it 24 hours after the baby becomes asymptomatic over a period of days (Appendix I). We have been doing this since June 1992 and have found that these babies have been made comfortable without being sedated and have consequently been able to feed. We have also been able to formulate a policy for the discharge of drug-dependent women and their babies, by following 104 babies born to opiate-dependent women who were on a methadone programme, up to 28 days of life. We found that babies who did not exhibit severe symptoms by 72 hours of age did not develop them later. Consequently they are discharged after this period, even if they have mild symptoms, if there are no medical reasons to keep them in hospital, provided that the mother is happy with this (Siney et al, 1995).

Although there is no easy way to predict withdrawal symptoms in neonates, in our five-year experience of almost 300 live births in the central Liverpool maternity service we have found that generally full-term healthy babies can cope well with withdrawal from quite large amounts of opiates and small weak babies find it difficult to cope with relatively small amounts of opiates. It would appear that problems with withdrawal depend on many variables including gestation and weight at delivery, the amount of opiates the mother has taken and when – in relation to labour – and the general condition of the baby. It would be easy to say that a large amount of opiate taken guarantees severe withdrawal symptoms in the neonate, and a small amount carries no risk, but this has not appeared to be the case in Liverpool. Matters can also be complicated by other drugs the mother may or may not admit to taking. Babies who have appeared not to exhibit obvious signs of withdrawal postnatally have often had episodes of distress in labour, shown by either meconium stained liquor or a sub optimal tracing on the cardiotocograph, and may even have had an operative or instrumental delivery because of 'fetal distress' which may have occurred due to withdrawal in the fetus during the course of labour. All opiate-dependent women who come into contact with the maternity/drug liaison service are told of the risks of neonatal withdrawal both during pregnancy and after birth and occasionally this has influenced a woman's decision to stop illicit opiate use and also reduce her methadone prescription in order to help the baby.

I think it is important to keep neonatal withdrawal in perspective – to ensure that babies who require treatment are given the right treatment, but equally that babies are not given treatment unnecessarily. Many babies exhibit some of the minor symptoms attributed to drug withdrawal (listed earlier) for all sorts of reasons, and they are not treated or sedated. Staff must be sure that symptoms are related to drug withdrawal before treatment is commenced and any reason other than drug withdrawal is excluded in the baby of an opiate-dependent woman.

The use of many score charts for observation of neonatal withdrawal is problematic, there is a risk of subjectivity. Many charts ask the observer if a symptom is mild or severe and allocates a score to it. Scores are added up and treatment is initiated when a certain score is reached. If an observer has never cared for an infant of a drug-dependent mother, can they decide on the severity of a symptom? If more than one observer is used over a period of time then how accurate is the observation? If an observer has certain views about drug misuse and pregnancy could this influence the observation? It would probably be more accurate to assess the well-being and need for treatment by looking at whether the baby is feeding and whether, even if agitated, he or she could be comforted enough to settle between feeds. The mother should be supported in her care of the baby so that her guilt and stress, and even the stress of the staff, do not influence the decision to treat the baby.

Antenatal HIV antibody testing

Drug misusers are often 'targeted' by maternity services (and indeed other health services) to offer testing for both HIV and hepatitis. If testing is to be offered on the basis of risk then it should be risk behaviour rather than risk group, and antenatal questioning for all women should reflect this. HIV testing was an issue for discussion and debate in 1987 at the Annual General Meetings of both the British Medical Association (BMA) and the Royal College of Midwives (RCM). The BMA decided that testing for HIV antibody should be at the discretion of the patient's doctor and should not necessarily require the consent of the patient, although it was later pointed out that taking blood for testing without consent was an assault in law and doctors were still ruled by their existing ethical standards. The RCM delegates voted against routine HIV antibody testing. November 1988 saw the Secretary of State for Health announce a major programme of anonymous prevalence testing for HIV. The UKCC published an information document in January 1989 which included advice to practitioners: that staff employed in places from which samples are obtained for prevalence testing were to be aware of this so that they could answer any questions asked; that patients or clients who objected to participation should not be discriminated against in any way or identified as being a higher risk than non-objectors or have required treatment withheld. This was reviewed in 1992, and again in 1993, with the issue of a Registrar's letter which gave the same advice (UKCC, 1989).

In 1990 the Institute of Medical Ethics working party published a report entitled *HIV Infection: The Ethics of Anonymized Testing and of Testing Pregnant Women.* It supported the view that explicit permission should normally be sought in the case of testing for HIV antibody. It discussed this in relation to anonymized HIV antibody testing for epidemiological purposes, concluding that this was to be welcomed given certain safeguards. It also argued that pregnant women may have a greater and more immediate need than others to know their HIV status, but concluded that this need did not justify testing them without their permission and should be met by voluntary diagnostic testing supported by adequate briefing (Boyd, 1990). (I think it is important here to comment that the temptation to view the pregnant woman merely as a host/carrier for a fetus should be resisted.)

In 1993 the Department of Health announced the latest results from the programme of anonymized surveys started in January 1990. The surveys provided information on the level of HIV infection in pregnant women, and people attending genito-urinary medicine (GUM) clinics and drug misuse centres, as well as from a pilot survey of people attending other clinical specialities in two London hospitals. The results confirmed the previous findings; for 1991 and the first half of 1992 the rates of HIV infection in pregnant women for inner and outer London were similar, remaining at 1:500. The rest of the country showed a rate of 1:16,000. At the end of 1992 the Department of Health issued guidance to providers of health care on offering voluntary named HIV antibody testing to women receiving antenatal care, as well as on establishing additional sites for HIV antibody testing (previously GUM clinics and drug misuse centres) and partner notification for HIV infection. Appendix 2 of this guidance stated, however, that the Department of Health wished to encourage the introduction of the policy of offering voluntary named HIV antibody testing to pregnant women in areas of known or suspected higher prevalence of HIV (Department of Health, 1992).

The issue of antenatal HIV antibody testing remains contentious but the UKCC guidance to nurses, midwives and health visitors remains the same as that issued in 1989. Practitioners must remember that blood and body fluids from all patients/clients pose a potential infection risk, and that HIV antibody testing (after counselling) is offered to women on the basis that it will be of benefit to them and not because it will make the staff feel more comfortable giving care. If practitioners perform care differently for people who they perceive to be at higher risk of HIV infection then there is something sadly amiss with their clinical practice; this, of course, does not mean that individualized plans of care for women are compromised.

Fetal rights versus maternal rights

Over the last few years a number of cases have arisen concerning fetal rights. There appears to be a trend to view maternal and fetal rights as antagonistic. The law relating to consent to treatment by the mentally competent adult is clear. If a patient/client refuses consent to treatment then any touching of that person is trespass. If the patient/client is unconscious then a doctor could act in an emergency to save her or his life as part of the doctor's duty of care to that patient. Consent does not need to be in writing to be legally effective, it can be given orally. The fact that a patient/client has come into hospital does not, however, imply consent to treatment.

A pregnant woman addicted to illicit drugs, alcohol or smoking tobacco, which was endangering the well-being of the fetus, would not be committing a criminal offence under the Infant Life (Preservation) Act 1929 unless there was evidence of intention of bringing about an abortion or destroying a child capable of being born alive. The 1929 Act makes it a criminal offence for 'any person who, with intent to destroy the life of a child capable of being born alive, by any wilful act, causes a child to die before it has an existence independent of its mother'. The only defence is preservation of the life of the mother. The Congenital Disabilities Act 1976 does not apply either. This Act was passed to give to the child born disabled as a result of a negligent act prior to its birth the right to sue in respect of that negligent act. It seems right that, provided health care professionals give all relevant information to a mother and also act in accordance with what is established practice, then the health care professionals cannot be deemed as negligent in law.

In the UK in 1985 the Social Services department in Berkshire obtained a 'place of safety order' (replaced in the Children Act 1989 by emergency protection orders) from Reading Juvenile Court and a baby girl, Victoria, was taken into care at a month old. While Victoria's mother – a registered drug addict – was pregnant she continued to take drugs in excess of those prescribed knowing that they could damage her child. Victoria was born prematurely, suffered from withdrawal symptoms, and was admitted to the special care baby unit where she remained for a number of weeks. In 1987 Victoria was still in foster care. Victoria's mother was never charged with any offence.

In 1986 in California a woman faced criminal charged arising from the death of her son. Thomas was born with massive brain damage after his mother started to haemorrhage slightly on 23 November 1985 at 0730 hours, and did not seek aid until 2000 hours that evening despite being told in her pregnancy that she had a placenta praevia condition, that she should not take unprescribed drugs, that she should rest, refrain from sexual intercourse and should seek medical aid if she started to haemorrhage. However, after starting to haemorrhage slightly she and her husband took some amphetamines and had sexual intercourse. She began to bleed more heavily and contractions began at 1400 hours. Thomas was born on 23 November 1985 with traces of amphetamine and marijuana in his blood; he died on 1 January 1987. His mother was charged under a section of the misdemeanour criminal code 1926 (USA). The statute makes it a crime for a parent to 'wilfully omit, without excuse, to furnish necessary medical attendance for her child'. Under this statute a fetus is deemed a person. This statute was designed to be used by women who seek support payments from husbands who have deserted them. The charges against Thomas' mother were dropped in March 1987 when the judge ruled that the 1926 law did not apply.

Arguments about mandatory treatment policies have gone on for a number of years in America and although both the American Medical Association and the American College of Obstetricians and Gynaecologists oppose mandatory treatment, in 1992 mandatory treatment policies existed in several states. Poor women and those from ethnic minorities are most often affected by them. A study of pregnant women in Florida by Dr Ira Chasnoff, Head of the Association for Perinatal Addiction Research, found that 14 per cent of black women and 15.4 per cent of white women used drugs, but 10 black women were reported for every white woman. The American Civil Liberties Union argues that forcing pregnant women to undergo treatment strips them of their rights (Tanne, 1991). In 81 per cent of the cases taken to court when a woman has refused treatment, the woman concerned has been a minority woman with a white male physician, and these statistics have been seen as a worrying trend by Mr

Lori Andrews, a research fellow of the American Bar Foundation and a senior scholar at the University of Chicago Centre for Medical Ethics. Women are usually charged with delivering drugs to a minor or under child abuse laws. Interestingly, in cases where women have been beaten by their partners and miscarried, no action was taken against the man (Tanne, 1992). It was reported in the British newspapers in August 1994 that a woman had been charged with murdering her child by breastfeeding him after snorting methamphetamine. This case is the first in America where a mother has been tried in this way, but this may create a precedent. Theoretically a mother drinking a few glasses of wine or smoking tobacco could be charged with the murder of her child if the child dies and a trace of alcohol or nicotine is found in its bloodstream. Should medical advice be given the status of law? If the fetus becomes a patient does the woman become merely the carrier? If women's choices about how they conduct their pregnancy and delivery are restricted then we may find that our ability as midwives to be supportive to women may be restricted too.

CHAPTER ONE

Management of Pregnant Women who are Drug-dependent

CATHERINE SINEY

Pregnancy outcomes in drug-dependent women have been reported for 20 years or more. The pregnancies of these women have always been regarded as 'high risk' both obstetrically and paediatrically. However it should be remembered that the majority, and earliest, of these outcome papers were and are from America, and in America the least advantaged and also the most needy people, have least access to healthcare. The links between infant and maternal mortality and poverty, poor health and nutrition are well documented and all the problems associated with drug misuse and dependence are also associated with social deprivation. There are many medical problems associated with heavy drug use, including anaemia and chronic bronchitis, and these and others are fully covered in the chapter on medical problems; other chapters cover human immunodeficiency virus (HIV), hepatitis and sexually transmitted diseases.

In general the main problems for the babies are intrauterine growth retardation, the risk of prematurity and, if the mother is opiate dependent, neonatal withdrawal problems. However acute withdrawal of opiates during pregnancy may precipitate enough distress in the fetus for spontaneous abortion or intrauterine death to occur. Indeed there are risks to the well-being of both mother and fetus of acute withdrawal from not only opiates but also barbiturates and benzodiazepenes. It is, therefore, essential that any antenatal care offered allows the woman to reduce these drugs of dependence slowly. Other drugs may usually just be stopped; maintenance of stimulant drugs, for example cocaine or tobacco, is inappropriate

Management of pregnancy in women who are drug-dependent must be holistic – this means not seeing these women as just a collection of problems but as women whose pregnancies are part of a larger picture of their lives, as indeed are all women's. Over the years great store has been set in pregnancy acting as a catalyst for women to stop misusing drugs but in our experience at the Liverpool Women's Hospital this has not proved to be the case in the majority of instances. In many cases, however, the lifestyles of women who were chaotic have become less so and many women already within a treatment programme have reduced their methadone or reduced/stopped the amount of illicit drugs they have used during their pregnancies. Some women have even managed to reduce their tobacco smoking. I think it is important that professionals involved with the pregnant woman should remember that, although all information about possible risks to the baby should be given, she should be supported in any attempts she makes to improve her health, and information should be given, and questions answered, in a non-judgmental way.

There have been programmes of maternity care involving a multidisciplinary approach since the 1970s in America and since the 1980s in the United Kingdom. A programme was started in the early 1970s in New York State which aimed to stabilize the women's life situation by offering a methadone programme and assistance to secure financial, legal and housing services. At the end of the first year 104 women had been referred to the programme and the conclusion drawn then was that a methadone programme, together with a great deal of psycho-social support, alleviated many of the common problems associated with drug dependence and pregnancy (Harper et al, 1974).

In the 1980s Fraser (1983) published a report on 72 pregnancies that had occurred between 1967 and 1982 describing their outcomes and concluding that management was complex with medical and social problems both during the pregnancy and afterward and he recommended an early case conference. Strang and Moran (1985), working in Manchester at the Regional Drug Dependence Unit, stressed the importance of combining antenatal care with a drug reduction programme and said that parenting skills should be judged by the same criteria applied to non-drug-dependent women. Dixon's article in *Druglink* (1987) gave a comprehensive view of the management of pregnant drug-dependent women from a social work perspective and concluded that each family situation should be looked at individually.

The 1990s have shown larger numbers of drug-dependent women having babies and much work, including papers by Dawe, Gerada and Strang (1992), Fraser and Cavanagh (1991) and Hepburn (1993), has talked of the importance of liaison and outreach services for female drug users.

Pre-conception care

General education about contraception to prevent unwanted pregnancy should be given to all women who enter treatment services or who have contact with outreach services (see chapters on 'The Sexual Health Needs of Female Drug Users' and 'Outreach Work with Female Sex Workers in Liverpool'). If pregnancy is planned then general health needs should be addressed, including rubella antibody screening, and any chronic medical problems should be discussed, including the effects on pregnancy and the fetus. For example, a number of the opiate dependent women seem to have no idea about their epileptic condition and the taking of anticonvulsants in pregnancy. The benefits of regular eating habits, a reduction in tobacco smoking and discussion about increased problems with constipation is useful. (Regular opiate use may affect bowel habits.)

Late booking

There are many reasons for late booking for hospital delivery. The problem of women not realizing they are pregnant till fetal movement is felt, or other physical changes occur, can be addressed by early contraceptive advice and access to pregnancy testing. For women who have no general practitioner (GP), the medical staff at the drug agencies should be able to refer pregnant women direct to an obstetrician, together with a letter with relevant drug history information. Women who are not in contact with drug agencies should be able to contact a specialist midwife at the maternity unit to access maternity care. In Liverpool information about the specialist midwife and the named consultants is distributed, by means of a poster (Appendix II) with a covering letter, to GPs by the Family Health Services Authority (FHSA), and to other relevant areas and departments.

The Liverpool service

Although pregnancies complicated by drug dependency are generally considered to be obstetrically 'high risk' it is often difficult to give them care at all. The Liverpool Women's Hospital has tried to operate a system of normalization for these women; we therefore decided that as long as the women were given antenatal care monthly by someone it did not really matter whether this was hospital care by an obstetrician or community care by a midwife or GP. The result has been that the women have accepted that monthly attendance somewhere for antenatal care is the minimum required to monitor the well-being of both themselves and their babies. Once women are known to the specialist midwife a bed booking is confirmed at the hospital. This means that even if the women do not attend the hospital until they are in labour, or have an antenatal problem, basic health, drug and social information is available, together with any follow-up antenatal visits by the specialist midwife, in the hospital records for the hospital staff.

Parent education

Parent education is offered to all women attending the hospital in the form of classes at different times of the day, including evenings; however it is also available on a one-to-one basis and for those women who are unable or do not wish to attend in the antenatal period then the parent education midwife visits the women on the ward in the postnatal period.

The general education includes information about the types of analgesia available in labour, an insight into the twenty four hour responsibility of parenting and basic instruction in bathing and infant feeding.

Screening and scans

An ultrasound scan for fetal anomalies is offered at 18 to 20 weeks, or at the first opportunity if the women enter the service after that, and is generally repeated only once unless there is a growth discrepancy. We thought at one time that ultrasound scans would attract the women to attend hospital more often but found that, although it worked occasionally to encourage the women to attend for the first scan, sometimes they would attend for ultrasound and then not carry on to the antenatal clinic appointment which followed. For those women not in touch with formal services the first ultrasound scan is usually arranged by the specialist midwife at the time she meets the women, by telephone if one is available, or a request form is left at the department and they are told that they can just turn up but will probably have to wait to be fitted in. However, whenever possible, if the women can give a time and day that will suit them then formal appointments are made.

Routine blood tests for blood grouping and antibodies, a full blood count and rubella antibodies are offered, but we also offer testing for hepatitis B surface antigen and antibodies and in 1994 we added testing for Hepatitis C. (Hepatitis B vaccination for the newborn baby is advised routinely if the women are Hepatitis B surface antigen positive during pregnancy.) Although HIV is discussed they are usually asked to discuss this further with their drug agency, if they have one, or the local Genito-Urinary Medicine department where full counselling and long term support facilities are available. Since the specialist midwife is available at the drug clinic/GP surgeries, either on a regular or ad hoc basis, HIV testing is discussed jointly on most occasions. Details of previous HIV tests are recorded in the hospital records only if the women wish it. A combined blood test to ascertain the level of risk of Down's Syndrome and open neural tube defects is offered to women if they are in time, that is between 15 and 20 weeks gestation. A specimen of urine is sent for screening for infection and care is taken to reassure the women that urine is never screened for drugs without the express permission of the women concerned.

Antenatal care

The antenatal care given by the specialist midwife, hospital obstetrician or GP surgery is the same care given to any pregnant woman. However, eating and tobacco smoking habits are discussed in detail because regular drug use may depress appetite and tobacco use may be much heavier in drug-dependent women. Also for those women who are prescribed injectable methadone or continue to inject illicit drugs during pregnancy it is important to know that they are using safe injection techniques and clean equipment. Women who usually inject into their groin may have problems as their stomachs enlarge; therefore, if they have no partner to inject for them, an alternative site needs to be suggested. Ideally, of course, injecting anything, whether prescribed or illicit, should be discouraged. We have had occasional problems with women injecting into breast veins and this can cause problems of mastitis and necrosis. (See Fig. 3.2 in Chapter Three, p.19.)

Drug treatment regime

The treatment regime for pregnant opiate dependent women by the local drug clinic – the Liverpool Drug Dependency Unit (LDDU) – is one of stabilization of opiate dependency on to an amount of daily methadone (either oral or for injecting, depending on what is appropriate for the woman) in the first trimester. Reduction is by a maximum of 5mgs at any one time in the middle trimester and a maintenance prescription in the last trimester. With women who are new into the local drug clinic as pregnant priority clients, the aim will be to stabilize drug use, and occasionally these women reduce their prescription during pregnancy. Clients already involved with the drug clinic may reduce their prescription if they are stable. However for some women, who come late in pregnancy into treatment, the aim will be to stabilize them. Some women will be able to reduce their prescription throughout the whole pregnancy and some women may have to have a small increase towards the end of the pregnancy. The women are always told of the possible risks of suddenly stopping opiates (and indeed barbiturates and benzodiazepenes) and if they want to stop we offer them either an in-patient maternity bed, or daily access to the fetal well-being unit, where the well-being of the fetus can be monitored, which ever is most appropriate. The LDDU works within a harm minimization framework, negotiating individual treatment plans with their service users. Urine testing is performed randomly at the clinic and they try not to test samples from the pregnant clients as a matter of course. The LDDU employs a female project worker who is able to pick up and transport women to and from appointments.

Women are always assured that methadone will be available to them, whether in a treatment programme or not, for any admission to hospital.

Social issues

It is essential for all professionals in contact with pregnant women who are drug-dependent to be assured that these women will be able to care adequately for their children when they go home from hospital. Because of the system of normalization within our hospital, the hospital social services department, the maternity liaison health visitor and the specialist midwife meet each month, or more often, to discuss all drug-dependent women known to the maternity service. Information is gathered from all professionals in contact with the women and the need for formal input or child protection conference is decided from this information. (The LDDU also have a regular meeting to discuss their pregnant clients and the social workers at the LDDU make any assessment needed.)

If a child protection conference is required for statutory reasons then this is usually arranged at least six weeks before the expected date of confinement. Having child protection conferences in advance of the delivery allows plans to be made and accepted and this in turn means that when the women deliver their babies the plans for child care are available to hospital staff in the hospital records. This enables the women and their babies to be discharged when obstetrically/paediatrically fit. Women and hospital staff generally have a happier time if everyone knows the plan and the hospital staff are able to reinforce the need for the women to comply with any agreed plan for child care.

Care in labour

All types of analgesia are available to the women in labour unless there is a medical contra-indication, for example, in the case of epidural analgesia the women must fulfil the safety criteria of the anaesthetist. Analgesia is given alongside the prescribed methadone – if a woman is not registered for treatment then the level of methadone needed to maintain the woman's comfort is assessed and given. We have found that opiate dependent women who have their methadone level maintained do not require any more analgesia in labour, or post-operatively, than other women.

Methadone is prescribed for the women as a daily dose so that they can ask for their medication at the usual time they take it and they can split up their medication as they would at home; also they may not actually require the full amount prescribed and they are reassured that their prescribing agency will not be told how much they have been asking for daily. The local drug prescribing agencies are well aware that their clients may vary their methadone dose. Injectable methadone is not available for in-patients in the hospital; this policy was agreed by the consultant in drug dependency at the LDDU, the obstetricians and the senior hospital pharmacist. During labour the fetus is monitored continually using a cardiotocograph. A paediatrician is usually present for the delivery, and after clinical assessment of the general condition of the baby, writes any instructions into the baby record. Many of the babies have proved to be growth retarded at birth and if so, then specific instructions regarding feeding may be required.

The use of naloxone hydrochloride for neonates (used to reverse opioid-induced respiratory depression) has been discontinued in our hospital following an audit by a paediatric consultant of the use of this drug in the delivery suite. It was felt that any benefit that there might be was outweighed by the risk that it might be given to the baby of an unknown opiate dependent woman and precipitate an acute opiate withdrawal crisis. It was a cause for concern since drug misuse in Liverpool is a large and growing problem and it seemed prudent to acknowledge this. Adult naloxone hydrochloride is available for use for resuscitation purposes.

Post-delivery care

Mothers and babies are cared for together within the postnatal area. Admission to the neonatal intensive care unit is for medical reasons only and not for observation. Babies are monitored four-hourly using the drug withdrawal chart (Appendix I). Symptoms are discussed at length during the antenatal period and the minimum length of time required for a postnatal stay, and this is discussed again after birth. Most women are distressed to see their babies suffering the effects of drug withdrawal and many are surprised when the degree is different from what they have been led to expect from other women. We try not to make the women feel any more guilty than they do already and give as much support as the women need to care for babies who may be difficult to settle. If treatment is required the babies stay with the mothers and the paediatricians and midwives spend time explaining what is happening and why the baby needs treatment. We try very hard not to make it seem like a punishment for their drug use. By treating neonatal opiate withdrawal as a paediatric medical problem and not a moral issue we have found that women are anxious for their babies to receive whatever treatment they require, and for as long as necessary. On very few occasions do women go home and leave their babies in hospital, only if a long stay in the neonatal unit is required. The urine or meconium of babies of drug-dependent women is not sent for drug screening; neither are the babies HIV tested. Any baby whose mother is found to be Hepatitis B surface antigen positive during pregnancy or labour is offered prophylactic Hepatitis B vaccination. We are constantly reviewing our care of the babies of drug-dependent women and have altered the neonatal drug withdrawal chart since the specialist service began in 1990. The chart currently in use is shown as Appendix I and the use of charts has been discussed in the earlier section 'Effects of drugs on pregnancy and the neonate'.

The midwives working in the community are notified when drug dependent women and their babies are discharged from hospital so that they can give them the support and reassurance they need. Babies are never discharged from hospital until the treatment with morphine sulphate has been completed. If babies show either no signs of withdrawal or only mild signs at 72 hours then they are discharged home once the mothers are happy that they can cope with the baby's needs. The health visitors are notified antenatally by the maternity liaison health visitor so that if the women are unknown to them they can visit and establish a contact before birth.

Future contraceptive needs are discussed during the antenatal period, in hospital and by the community staff, and if female sterilization is an option then an appointment is made for a later date to discuss this.

Aims of the specialist service

The aims of the service have been to normalize the care of pregnant drug-dependent women, to make it an attractive, easily accessible service and one that gives them a positive birth experience. The service has proved to be accessible with increased numbers of women approaching either before their pregnancies or earlier in their pregnancies and it has also reduced the ratio of drug-dependent women arriving unbooked and in labour.

Training for staff

Twice yearly the specialist midwife organizes lectures/workshops to discuss drugs and pregnancy for all grades of staff. It is hoped that staff will not only gain information from these sessions but will also look at their attitudes so that they can ensure that all women in their care receive the care they are entitled to without fear of bias. The hospital is constantly reviewing clinical practice to ensure the safety of all patients and staff. Information about clinical management and social support is available to all staff in all departments (Appendix III).

CHAPTER TWO

Women and Drug Use

SUE RUBEN

Drug misuse treatment with particular reference to women

Illegal drug use has increased markedly all over the world. Treatment agencies are generally predominated with treating male drug misusers and, although it appears that the overall number of women is lower than men, there is considerable evidence to suggest that the number of women using and experiencing severe problems with illegal drug use is increasing. Women are often reluctant to take advantage of treatments that are available to them.

The social stigma around drug use is probably more for women than men as it very much goes against their perceived role as carers and the perception that they should in some way be more responsible than men. In common with alcohol use in women, drug taking is often hidden. Women experience extreme guilt and fear the consequences of admitting the problem as they are very concerned that this will have worse consequences with particular regard to their children than trying to cope without expert help. Professionals therefore need to take seriously the particular issues for women and try to ensure that services for drug users take account of women's needs and fears, working with their women users to overcome prejudice.

Why do women misuse drugs?

Women who become problematic drug users may do so for a huge variety of reasons. They are often introduced to drugs by drug-taking sexual partners who at times see no problem in their own drug use but are extremely critical of the woman when she follows their lead.

Drug taking may be used to alleviate stress, anxiety and depression or may be entered into initially as a recreational activity without recognizing the serious consequences that may ensue. In my experience the veins of women seem not to withstand injecting for as long as their male counterparts and they often run into early problems with injection sites.

Women with children are in constant fear that if they admit their problem, their children will be taken into care by social workers. It is therefore imperative that drug services look to reducing this as a consequence and work closely with local social services departments to ensure that systems can be put in place which reduce this possibility.

Clearly there cannot be a blanket statement that no woman drug user will have their child removed as under the Children's Act the care of the child and its needs are paramount. However, statements such as the one that drug use *per se* is not a reason for removing children and that every opportunity will be used to try and keep children with their drug-using mothers, can realistically help in reassuring women. One would hope that, in good treatment facilities, women who are accepting their problems and working towards solving them in a positive way would be less likely to experience child care problems than those who are not in touch with treatment, and this needs to be constantly striven for.

Services need to be aware of the ways in which women obtain money to sustain a drug habit. Prostitution has increasingly become a mode of obtaining money to buy drugs and this in itself causes major problems for women. Firstly prostitution is an extremely risky profession. The woman is at risk from a health point of view with regard to sexually transmitted diseases, HIV and Hepatitis B (these will be dealt with in other chapters). They are also at risk of physical abuse by their clients. The work is often done in unsafe places such as red light districts in cities and, in order to overcome their distaste for prostitution, many women find that their drug use escalates out of control faster than before they resorted to prostitution. This can lead to a rapid down-spiralling in terms of their abilities to cope and survive. While it is relatively easy to earn money as a prostitute, if the drug use escalates this clearly does not help the individual to survive in a safe way within our modern society.

Once women enter into the criminal justice system, this again tends to have very serious negative effects with regard to their family relationships and care for their children. Whereas men going to prison, for example, can usually rely on women left outside to continue with parental roles and child rearing, this is often not an option for women and is extremely disruptive to any possibility of them parenting their children successfully.

Treatment

Treatment of women drug users, in my view, requires a multidisciplinary approach with a range of input from interested professionals. Often it is not simply that they have problems with drug use in their lives but have a multitude of social, emotional and financial difficulties with associated chronic low self-esteem. All these aspects of their life need to be tackled if they are either to overcome their drug problem or benefit from substitution treatments such as methadone. Interventions need to take account of the individual's particular needs and deficits and aim to work with the woman in a positive way. They should always emphasize what can be done and how they can again take control of their life while recognizing that helping any individual with a drug problem can be a time-consuming business. The natural history of serious drugs misuse is that it is a recurring condition with periods of relative stability and it is easy to fall back into more problematic use with its attendant consequences.

This again puts women under particular pressures and it is during periods of chaos when their social problems and inability to care adequately for children may cause yet more stress and difficulties for them.

The first thing to be tackled by treatment agencies is ensuring that women have ready access into treatment. This can be relatively successfully helped by, for example, the use of specific outreach workers with female drug users, in particular female prostitutes. They can be the important first link for a woman into the helping system. As well as giving high quality advice on the spread of sexually transmitted diseases, HIV and Hepatitis, they can encourage women to take up a treatment option and, if need be, accompany them to an appointment. Treatment agencies need to educate social services and primary health care teams in considering drug misuse in women who are having particular problems in coping.

Treatment agencies can ensure that their facility is welcoming for women by having an area with toys for children to play with, baby changing facilities and leaflets that particularly emphasize women's issues, to ensure that women do not feel ostracized or criticized by seeking help. Agencies should constantly be monitoring their referral patterns to ensure that women are being referred and, if not, they should take active steps to encourage referrals.

It is worth having particular staff members take a clear interest in women and their particular problems and introducing women drug users to them early on in treatment. We have found in Liverpool that the policy of prioritizing female prostitutes and pregnant users into the methadone programme has been very helpful in encouraging women to come forward for help and treatment.

In my experience the treatment options which might be offered to a woman are no different than those that could be offered to any drug user regardless of sex. However particular attention may be needed to ensure that women can take advantage of treatment facilities and are able to keep regular appointments with the drug clinic team. It is pointless giving women with children appointments which clash with school times and it may be more appropriate to try and offer a lot of the support in the person's own home, if this can be arranged and the woman is agreeable.

The philosophy of harm minimization

It is my belief that the sort of interventions that are available for drug users should fall broadly within a philosophy of harm minimization. By that I mean that all interventions offered to people should have an objective of reducing the harm that their drug-taking behaviour is causing both to them as individuals and also to their family and the community as a whole.

The overall aim of any harm minimization programme should be to ultimately for people to lead a drug-free life and be self-supporting in their community. It also has to be recognized that this is often an unrealistic initial goal for people and the intermediary goals are worth aiming for on the way to a drug-free life. We must acknowledge that not all individuals are going to achieve the ultimate goal but if they manage improvements in their social stability, general health, injecting behaviour and ability to care for their children, this in itself is positive and worth achieving.

Consideration has to be given, of course, to the treatment options depending on the drug or drugs used by women. In general, women's drug use reflects the pattern of drug use in the community in which the woman lives. In the UK in the present time it is still true to say that the most common problematic illegal drug is heroin. However drugs such as the stimulants cocaine and amphetamines are commonly used and minor tranquilizers, particularly benzodiazepenes, are commonly misused. The dangers of the abuse of sleeping preparations such as temazepam cannot be over-emphasized. It is also well known that women are more likely to be prescribed benzodiazepene than men and therefore benzodiazepene abuse is extremely common in this group.

Many women are what is known as 'polydrug abusers' in that they use and abuse more than one class of drug. All this has to be taken account of in the initial assessment period. At the first assessment a decision needs to be made as to whether any form of prescription is likely to assist or whether the individual should be helped by counselling, support and other forms of intervention, such as a rapid detoxification programme.

Oral methadone

Experience has shown that the people who are highly dependent on opiate-class drugs tend to benefit from a period of stabilization on an opiate substitute. In the UK the most commonly prescribed drug for this purpose is oral methadone. Oral methadone has major advantages; firstly it is well absorbed orally and has been shown consistently to reduce injecting behaviours. Secondly it is a long-acting drug and can therefore be taken on a once-daily or twice-daily basis. This stabilizes the individual's mental state and can enable them, with assistance, to start planning and organizing their life in a more appropriate and positive manner. It has to be recognized that methadone is itself an opiate drug and therefore highly addictive. It therefore does not cure addiction but can enable an unstable addict to become a stable addict with a legal prescription and with no drug-related need to resort to criminal activity. It also enables the person to work on other aspects of their life.

Many women have poor coping skills and strategies and need considerable assistance with things such as managing money, caring for children, health care and developing social skills. My experience is that the input of people such as specialist health visitors and social workers can be invaluable in assisting the woman to organize herself and her family more successfully while she is on a prescription.

During treatment with methadone urine testing can form part of a vital strategy for monitoring the individual's drug use on top of their prescription. It gives workers a way of monitoring progress and it can, if used properly, help the drug user to stabilize their own life. Usually it has been found that on methadone programmes the use of other drugs on top of the prescription significantly reduces and around 50 per cent of people can be expected over time to stop altogether. While it is clearly desirable that, wherever possible, methadone prescription should be for as short a time as possible, experience has shown that for some individuals who are attempting to stabilize other aspects of their life, the prescription may be for a longer time than would have initially been desirable. This should not be seen as failure but rather as an inevitable consequence of trying to help individuals with very many social and other problems.

The most important thing in a successful methadone programme appears to be a good working relationship between the drug user and the staff on that programme. It is essential to encourage people to be honest and open with the staff while reassuring them that they will not be punished for honesty.

Inpatient detoxification

For other female drug users it may be more appropriate to consider a period of inpatient detoxification. This means that the team must ensure that adequate provision has been made for any children of the woman, so that while she is in hospital the children are well cared for. Strenuous efforts have to be made to ensure that the children can visit their mother whilst she is in hospital and that the children have themselves appropriate support so that they can cope without their mother, who they may indeed be very anxious about, particularly if they have been aware that she has not been well and have not been aware of the reason for her behaviour towards them.

Once successfully detoxified, it is absolutely vital that appropriate aftercare is organized for the woman and her family. This may take the form of opiate-antagonist drugs such as naltrexone and appropriate support/counselling and training opportunities also seem to be vital during this time.

For a small proportion of women, longer term rehabilitation in family units away from her usual community may be required. There is a very small number of such units within the UK and the costs often prove prohibitive as these currently have to be met by overstretched social services monies for care in the community and some programmes last for up to 12 months.

I have tried therefore to emphasize the positive gains that can be offered to women drug users, their particular difficulties and some general ways in which the needs of women as service users must be addressed. Individuals working with women drug users need to examine their own attitudes and take into account the fact that these may adversely affect a woman in treatment, and all multidisciplinary teams need to constantly review and reassess the particular needs of their women drug users as they arise.

About the author

Dr Susan M. Ruben is Clinical Director for the Drugs and HIV Prevention Directorate for the North Mersey Community (NHS) Trust. She qualified at Edinburgh University in 1978.

Dr Ruben is a member of the Royal College of Psychiatrists. She has specialized in drug misuse for the last eight years and is on the Executive Committee of the Substance Misuse Section of the College and a member of the Advisory Council on the Misuse of Drugs. In 1994 Dr Ruben was *Liverpool Echo*'s 'Mum of the Year'.

CHAPTER THREE

The Medical Problems of Illicit Drug Misuse in Pregnancy and Harm Minimization

CLIVE L. MORRISON

The misuse of drugs, particularly the injecting misuse, carries with it a considerable mortality and morbidity. Often users hide their problems for fear of being discovered as an addict. Judgmental attitudes towards drug users from health care staff also prevents users gaining access to the normal emergency medical services from casualty and general practice. This tends to make problems, which would have easily been resolved with simple treatments if presented earlier, more problematic when it appears that the user has neglected her condition. In reality it is the health services that have excluded her from care.

The problems of drug misuse affect men and women equally, but when a woman is pregnant issues become more emotive and rather than being seen as an individual, who can exercise the right to lead her own lifestyle, she is treated more as a 'baby machine' with problems not only considered as self-inflicted but also as harmful to her pregnancy. These effects are largely related to the illegal nature of drugs and having no access to needle and syringe exchanges. Having clean needles and syringes and receiving safer drug use advice from drug agencies within a harm minimization framework reduces the problems of drug misuse. However, misusers can still encounter accidental overdosage, withdrawal symptoms, cardiac and pulmonary problems, dental caries, abscesses, cellulitis, endocarditis, septicaemia, viral Hepatitis, genito-urinary infections and HIV (some of these aspects are covered in other chapters).

Overdosage and withdrawal

One of the problems of illicit drug use is that users obtain irregular supplies from the illegal market. Concentrations of the drug can vary even from the supplier depending upon how much the drug is cut down with adulterants. The higher the profit motive the more the drug will be diluted along the chain of supply. If a woman has been used to injecting a certain supply which then becomes more concentrated, then there is a potential to overdose. Opiate overdose requires immediate hospitalization to monitor any respiratory suppression and also to prevent asphyxiation after vomiting. The opiate antagonist, naloxone, when administered usually brings a quick recover. Pulmonary oedema is one of the most common and serious effects of heroin overdose. Some far-sighted agencies instruct users in life support techniques that could be used if an acquaintance succumbs to overdosage, whilst waiting for the ambulance. Radical proposals have suggested that drug users should be issued with naloxone ampoules that they could inject as required. However, it is believed that naloxone would be too dangerous to use outside of hospital and pregnant women would certainly need adequate fetal monitoring.

The misuse of tricyclic anti-depressants, cocaine and cyclizine can cause cardiac arythmias and, when this causes sudden death, it is usually considered as an overdose. It has been estimated that around one per cent of injecting drug users die each year this way. At the other end of the spectrum is withdrawal which in pregnancy can cause miscarriage in the first trimester, fetal compromise and premature labour in the final trimester.

The symptoms of opiate withdrawal in the adult include, rhinorrhoea, lachrymation, abdominal cramps, gooseflesh, diarrhoea, muscle cramps and insomnia. Opiates are the only illicit drugs that cause a physical dependence and there is no adult morbidity associated with opiate withdrawal. Opiate withdrawal can be managed easily by using the oral substitute methadone. The amount used can be titrated according to the suggested table below.

Table 3.1: Methadone equivalents for drug of dependence

Drug	Dose	Methadone equivalent
Street Heroin	1/4 g	20 mg[1]
Pharmaceutical Heroin	30 mg ampoule	50 mg
Dipipanone	10 mg	4 mg
Codeine Phosphate	30 mg	2 mg
Dihydrocodeine	30 mg	3 mg
Dextromoramide	10 mg	10-20 mg
Buprenorphine	200 mcg	5 mg
Codeine Linctus	100 ml'	10 mg

[1]*Dose varies according to purity available in the community. Drug services will have the appropriate experience to titrate according to the local illicit supply.*

In areas where there are well-developed drug treatment agencies, the obstetric services should not involve themselves with the intricacies of methadone prescribing and should seek at all times the advice of their health care colleagues, hopefully within the structure of an obstetric liaison service.

The other illicit drugs such as cocaine, amphetamines or LSD do not create any physical dependence. The psychological dependency to these drugs can be considerable but there are no physical symptoms associated with abrupt withdrawal, or any evidence of harm to the fetus.

Dental hygiene

In any group of observed drug misusers on methadone there is a high rate of dental caries. Generally users have poor individual dental hygiene care and blame the high sugar content of methadone mixture, but there has been no research to make any conclusions on this. Again users have difficulty in accessing dental care due to dentists' fears of cross infection, but the level of anxiety related to dental treatment is still as high as the general population, even though drug misusers may be injectors themselves. As a consequence of multiple dental caries, dental abscesses are common. A thorough dental assessment with appropriate referral should be performed at the appointment for booking antenatal care. Poor dental hygiene allows for the copious growth of anaerobes in oral secretions and these are commonly involved in aspiration pneumonia. Symptoms may be only minor and present for many weeks. Eventually lung abscesses may form but these may not show on x-ray until a cavity lesion is present.

Respiratory system problems

Pulmonary vascular granulomatosis can occur in injecting drug users when they inject crushed tablets such as dipipanone and methadone that are intended for oral use. The granulomas are an immune reaction to the talc that is used in tablets to bulk and carry the active drug. The illness presents as progressively increasing shortness of breath in association with a productive cough. These symptoms can also occur in heroin use, when the adulterants in the drug can embolize to the lung, including fibres from cigarette filters, which are commonly used by drug users to filter out residue when preparing heroin to inject.

Pieces of needles being used to inject drugs can break off, particularly in very fibrous injecting sites and embolize to the lung but these are best treated consecutively.

Research in the United States suggests that the incidence of tubercular disease in drug users is higher than the general population due to factors related to lifestyle such as poor nutrition, close contact and depressed state of health due to other infections. In New York 20 per cent of drug users had positive screening tests for TB. Some drug treatment agencies have added prophylactic anti-tubercular chemotherapy into the oral methadone to such drug users. However in the UK public health and social policies are completely different, with the school BCG vaccination programme and welfare limiting poverty to some extent. There is no such association with drug users and TB in this country other than for social class.

Inhaling the fumes of heroin can also be problematic. The drug releases histamine and this process can produce asthma. The snorting of cocaine can damage the cartilage between the nostrils and produce a perforation. Snorting any drug can increase the incidence of rhinorrhoea, allergic rhinitis and infected sinuses.

Injecting drug users are more likely to acquire chest infections than the general population. The risk is ten times greater but the infection responds well to the usual treatments. Pulmonary fungal infection has occurred, the cause being identified as due to the presence of candida albicans in lemon juice. This is used to acidify and to help the solution to dissolve illicit heroin, to render it injectable.

Subcutaneous, deep, mycotic and septicaemic infections

Local skin infections are the most common presentation in injecting drug misusers. This clinical problem ranges from small abscesses, cellulitis, thrombophlebitis to necrotizing fascitis. The predominant organisms isolated from such infections are usually staphylococci and streptococci. Infections that remain localized without systemic effects can be treated with either magnesium sulphate dressings at an early stage or, if the abscess is pointing, then incised and drained. The antibiotics of choice are either flucloxacillin or clindamycin, which are active against the most common organisms and have good soft tissue penetration.

Women do not have as well-developed veins as men on their peripheral limbs. Therefore, injecting is more difficult and when there is no further venous access some women resort to skin popping. The trauma of repeated injecting into the subcutaneous tissues can cause ulcers and low grade infection (Fig. 3.1).

During pregnancy the veins in women do become more prominent due to higher circulating hormone levels with the breast veins developing more so. The breast veins are unable to tolerate venepuncture and become easily infected or the puncture site becomes necrotic (Fig. 3.2).

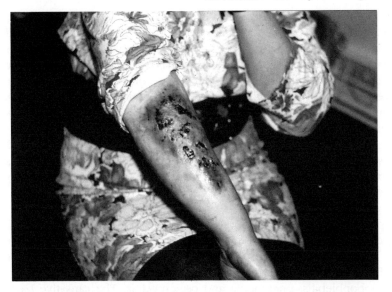

Fig. 3.1: Effects of repeated injection into subcutaneous tissues

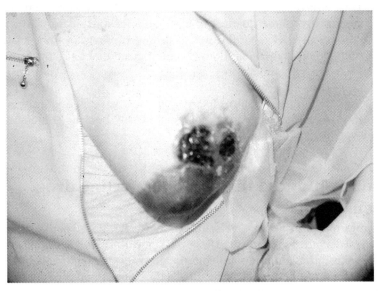

Fig. 3.2: Breast abscess due to injecting

Skin necrosis with super infection can occur with extravazation of the injected drug into the surrounding tissues. This can lead on to the most serious of subcutaneous infections, necrotizing fascitis.

More serious infections require hospitalization with culturing of swab taken from site of the infected area. Blood cultures should also be taken before the commencement of intravenous antibiotics.

Subcutaneous infection can cause septic emboli which result in septic pulmonary infarcts. When this condition co-exists with endocarditis, mortality can be up to 16 per cent. The tricuspid value is most frequently affected in drug misusers and the organism is usually staphylococcus aureus. There should always be a high index of suspicion of endocarditis in an injecting drug user who has a fever, even without the classical evidence of a murmur or any local infected sites. There are very few drug users who can tolerate the six-week course of antibiotics and many discontinue this regime, being discharged on oral antibiotics. Valve replacement should be advised in those users with congestive cardiac failure, continual sepsis or repeated embolism, but would not be of any benefit in those who would continue to inject illicit drugs.

Septicaemia is cased by endocarditis in 40 per cent of cases in drug users. The majority occurs as a result of soft tissue infection with the groin area around the femoral vein – the most common site of primary infection. Other less common causes are mycotic aneurysms, septic arthritis, thrombophlebitis, pneumonia and osteomyelitis. The causative bacteria are staphylococcus aureus and group A streptococci. Osteomyelitis occurs in injecting drug users by haematogenous seeding. Pseudomonas aeruginosa accounts for over three quarters of all bone infections, mainly involving the vertebrae and pelvic girdle. Septic arthritis presents as a hot, swollen and painful joint on moving. Both require regular antibiotics over several weeks to resolve the infection.

Injecting drug users should ensure that they have adequate tetanus protection, as injecting paraphernalia could easily become contaminated in unhygienic conditions.

Trauma-induced injury from injecting drug misuse

Injecting into arm veins classically produces the 'track' marks running down the length of the forearm. However, some users who have obliterated these veins through thrombophlebitis begin to use the femoral vein in the groin. Scars on the arms can heal over time and it could easily appear from a cursory medical examination that the user was not injecting. Looking more carefully at the groin site will either show granulation tissue in someone who has only just begun injecting there but this will eventually break down to leave a sinus communicating to the femoral vein. Constant use of this site invariably leads to the formation of a deep venous thrombosis (DVT), although the risk is substantially increased if gel-filled temazepam capsules are used as these can resolidify within the femoral vein. DVT is the most common emergency hospital referral from the Maryland Centre.

Treatment commences with heparin initially until the diagnosis is confirmed when the anti-coagulation therapy is changed to warfarin. A DVT presents with an intensely painful swollen leg and can be associated with pitting oedema. The aim of treatment is to prevent a fatal pulmonary embolism, although users are more concerned that their leg is the more serious problem, which resolves on rest, analgesics and graduated support stockings. Long-term warfarin therapy can prove to be difficult in those with chaotic lifestyles and should be discontinued in those who continue to inject. Heparin would be used throughout the length of a pregnancy.

In those who have had recurrent bilateral DVTs, femoral vein areas may not be present and some women have used their femoral artery to continue injecting. Repeated puncture with a needle causes an aneurysm which, if discovered, requires emergency vascular surgery. This type of injecting has associated with it a particular syndrome when temazepam is misused. 'Temazepam leg' is either caused by an allergic reaction to the temazepam capsule residue causing a vasculitis followed by secondary thrombosis or the small arterioles are blocked by micro-emboli rendering areas of muscle ischaemia. This in turn produces massive rhabdomyolysis which can affect renal function. If fasciotomy is unsuccessful in treating the associated compartment syndrome the user will require amputation.

The use of other central venous sites such as subclavicular and supraclavicular veins can cause tension pneumothoraces, haemothoraces or pyopneumothoraces. Loss of the function of the voice has been reported after damage to the vagus or recurrent laryngeal nerves near the site of injection.

Harm minimization

Harm minimization is a health and social policy which prioritizes the aim of decreasing the problems of drug misuse. Reducing these effects on health can be difficult as drugs are illegal and their use covert, and in some drug users the risks of criminal activity to fund their own drug use are more paramount to them than the considerable risks they take with their health.

Total abstinence is not an option for a majority of users who wish to continue taking drugs for whatever reason. Ensuring that they are able to use drugs in a safer manner protects the individual and society. The UK Government's response to the advent of HIV was expressed by the Advisory Committee on Drugs Misuse in 1988 who recommended a hierarchy of goals in harm minimization.

1.   The cessation of sharing of injecting equipment.
2.   A move away from injectable to oral drug use.
3.   A reduction in the quantity of drugs consumed.
4.   Abstinence.

The first goal was achieved by the opening of Needle and Syringe Exchanges (NSE) in 1986. These schemes aim to reduce the need to share injection equipment so limiting the spread of the viral transmissible diseases HIV and Hepatitis B. Clean and sterile injecting equipment helps protect the individual user and also the community within which they live. NSEs also provide for the safe disposal of contaminated equipment and injecting paraphernalia, information on HIV and sexual health matters, free condoms and referral to drug treatment agencies. Some similar to the Maryland Centre offer primary health care and safer drug use advice.

Some problems related to the injecting use of drugs are due to poor technique. Users are advised to use a quick release tourniquet which must be released after venepuncturing a suitable vein and before injecting the drug. Some users do not clean their skin prior to injecting or use saliva, and so alcohol wipes are issued. The licking of needles to remove subcutaneous fat tissues after an unsuccessful attempt to venepuncture is discouraged. Users are instructed on the appropriate size of needle to use and to inject in the direction of the flow of blood. Some users repeatedly fill their syringes with blood in the expectation that they are ensuring all the drug is injected (flushing) but this generally leads to loss of blood around the vessel, leading to fibrosis and phlebitis and so reducing the available veins for further access.

It is hoped that regular contact with NSE staff encourages beneficial behavioural change and facilitates the earlier contact with drug treatment agencies, so shortening the length of time a user is on illicit drugs.

The other goals in harm minimization are addressed by drug rehabilitation and treatment programmes. Originally the provision of methadone maintenance programmes was limited within the UK with users in some regions having no access to methadone whatsoever. The situation has improved to such an extent now that there is generally a service prescribing methadone within a district of England and Wales.

About the author
Dr Clive L. Morrison is a vocational trained General Practitioner and has worked for four years in substance misuse and HIV prevention. In his role as Senior Clinical Medical Officer for Special Groups he provides family

health care for drug users, prostitutes and HIV positive people. He has a unique expertise in the management of the complications of injecting drug misuse.

He has a special interest in the care and prescribing of methadone to pregnant drug users within the Liverpool Drug Dependency Clinic. Another role is to liaise between the local GUM and Drug Dependency services. He has collaborated in many research projects with other allied health professionals including the Regional Infectious Diseases Unit with a particular emphasis on the health care needs of drug users.

CHAPTER FOUR

Obstetric Problems for Drug Users

COLETTE SPAREY AND STEVE WALKINSHAW

The incidence of drug misuse has been rising for some time, with particular bursts of increase occurring at the beginning of each of the last three decades (Ministerial Group on the Misuse of Drugs, 1988). Information regarding drug misuse is often difficult to obtain with any accuracy, the illegality of both the possession and use of these substances making people unwilling to admit to their habits. Nevertheless, the number of registered heroin addicts increased by 21 per cent between 1991 and 1992.

In recent years there has been a change in the type of drugs misused with a move away from heroin towards the use of pharmaceutical products and poly-drug use (Hepburn, 1992). Drug misuse has increased disproportionately in women and is now almost equal to that in the male population and, thus, since the majority of drug abusers are young (i.e. in their teens and twenties), a substantial number of the drug misusers will be women of childbearing age.

Although the socio-economic background and lifestyle of these women is not specific to pregnancy, consequences may be expected. For example, they may be socially isolated and have housing, economic or domestic problems. Their lifestyle is often chaotic as attempts to finance and feed their habit can result in self-neglect and poor diet and may cause them to resort to prostitution and petty crimes to fund drug use (It is estimated that the average heroin addict gets through £30,000 worth of heroin per annum). Prostitution and other criminal activity not only have legal implications but, in the case of the former, have serious implications for the woman's health with 'side effects' ranging from sexually-transmitted diseases such as gonorrhoea, chlamydia, Hepatitis B and HIV infection to the risk of physical violence.

However dismal the potential picture, it is important to remember that many drug users lead perfectly normal lives, some holding down a job, many running a family and the majority differing little from their non drug-using peers (Ministerial Group on the Misuse of Drugs, 1988).

In the following pages some of the impact of drug misuse in pregnancy is outlined.

Opiates

The opiates most commonly used are heroin (diacetylmorphine) and methadone. Heroin is derived from morphine, a naturally occurring opiate found in the poppy, *papaver somniferum*, whilst methadone is a synthetic drug. Heroin is more soluble than most other opiates and is therefore absorbed more rapidly into the central nervous system giving a quicker and more intense 'high' to the user, hence it is the drug of choice for most addicts. Methadone on the other hand is more slowly absorbed, has a longer half life and thus produces more stable blood levels, making it a suitable drug for treating addicts who are trying to 'kick the habit'.

Maternal effects

Amenorrhoea is common among opiate addicts, possibly mediated through a decreased production of gonadotrophins. Accurate dating of the pregnancy is therefore difficult, not only because of the irregular menstrual cycle but also because these women tend to book late in pregnancy, if at all. At these stages even ultrasound dating will be inaccurate.

Nutrition amongst addicts is poor and thus anaemia and various vitamin deficiencies, including B6, folate and thiamine, are common. This problem is often aggravated during the first trimester by hyperemesis which may persist throughout pregnancy.

Opiate addicts who are using the drug intravenously will be at risk or a variety of unusual infections including bacterial endocarditis, thrombophlebitis, pneumonia, bronchitis and, if sharing needles, there is the risk of Hepatitis B and HIV infection. Both past and current intravenous use of drugs may affect maternal venous access. Thrombosis of peripheral veins, caused by repeated intravenous injection of impure heroin and possibly by the use of dirty needles causing infective thrombophlebitis, makes the insertion of cannulae and the taking of blood for investigations difficult if not impossible. Another 'side effect' of prolonged opiate abuse is tolerance to its effects which, in the context of pregnancy and labour is most relevant to its analgesic qualities. Much higher doses are necessary during labour to achieve the same effect as in a non drug user; alternatively epidural analgesia may be an option since this will be as effective as in the general population.

Fetal effects

The incidence of multiple pregnancies is thought to be increased although the exact mechanism is unknown. It may be related to a direct effect of opiates on ovarian function, causing dizygotic twinning. The incidence of congenital malformations is not increased by the use of opiates alone, before or during pregnancy.

Problems specific to pregnancy include an increased risk of antepartum haemorrhage due both to abruptio placentae and placenta praevea. The incidence of gestational hypertension and breech presentation are also reported to be increased (Silver et al, 1987; Finnegan, 1982). Whether these complications are a specific effect of opiates or more a reflection of the woman's general health and socio-economic circumstances is difficult to ascertain. The two most consistently reported findings are of a higher incidence of preterm deliveries and small-for-gestational-age babies (Thornton et al, 1990; Chasnoff et al, 1986; Kaltenbach and Finnegan, 1987; Klenka, 1986; Perlmutter, 1974; Ellwood et al, 1987; Gregg et al, 1988), up to 20 per cent in some series. Most studies also report an increase in intrauterine and neonatal deaths (Blinick et al, 1976; Perlmutter, 1974; Fricker and Segal, 1978; Finnegan, 1982). Intrauterine deaths may be related to repeated episodes of withdrawal caused by the erratic drug consumption by the mother. These episodes lead to intrauterine hypoxia which, if severe, results in intrauterine death. However, recent evidence in acute withdrawal programmes does not support this (Hepburn and Forrest, 1988). The aetiology of the increase in preterm labour is unclear. It may be related to increases in genital infection, a well established case of preterm labour (Salafia et al, 1991; Schwartz et al, 1989; Armer and Duff, 1991; Krohn et al, 1991; McGregor et al, 1991; McDonald et al, 1991) and therefore closely linked with lifestyle.

Fetal assessment may be difficult since opiates are known to alter non-stress tests by reducing baseline variability and causing loss of accelerations. Opiates also suppress fetal breathing movements; thus whether these findings are drug related or an indication of genuine fetal compromise is difficult to deduce in the individual case. Fetal movements are also affected by opiates in particular; withdrawal causes an increase in fetal activity about 30 minutes after the onset of maternal symptoms (Robins et al, 1993). Considerable care needs to be exercised in labour, if prolonged, as withdrawal of the woman's normal opiate dose may provoke fetal withdrawal and unusual fetal heart rate patterns.

Neonatal effects

The effects of maternal opiate addiction on the newborn and infant need to be considered. Apart from the complications of preterm delivery and low birthweight to which these neonates are more prone, there is the risk of Neonatal Abstinence Syndrome (NAS), or withdrawal. The symptoms to be looked out for are listed here.

- Tremor
- Sweating
- Irritability
- Fever

- High pitched cry
- Sneezing
- Respiratory distress
- Hyperactivity

- Vomiting
- Convulsions
- Hypertonicity
- Diarrhoea

The majority of symptoms appear within 24 to 48 hours of birth but have been reported up to six days after delivery (Perlmutter, 1974). Whether the onset, severity or duration of NAS is loosely related to the dose of opiate taken by the mother is uncertain. Some studies have found no correlation (Fricker and Segal, 1978; Mack et al, 1991) while others find the opposite (Strauss et al, 1974; Dobenczak et al, 1991; Harper et al, 1977). Methadone can cause more severe and prolonged withdrawal symptoms and delayed reactions may be more common (Perlmutter, 1974; Strauss et al, 1974; Blinick et al, 1976). If taken in conjunction with diazepam the onset of symptoms may again be delayed (Sutton and Hinterliter, 1990).

The risk of Sudden Infant Death Syndrome is five times greater in this group of infants (Rajegouda et al, 1978; Ellwood et al, 1987). Developmental delay may be more common (Oroffson et al, 1983) and there is the risk of being orphaned by maternal death due to either accidental or deliberate overdose, infection including HIV/AIDS or trauma.

Cocaine

Cocaine is an alkaloid derived from the coca plant. The water-soluble salt form can be absorbed through any mucosal surface (e.g. 'snorting') while a free cocaine base, 'crack', can be smoked, the latter being highly addictive and dangerous. The drug is a powerful vasoconstrictor and has been reported to be associated with maternal hypertension, spontaneous abortion and placental abruption (Chasnoff et al, 1985; Smith and Deitch, 1987; Acker et al, 1983; Macgregor et al, 1987). It has also been reported to be associated with small-for-gestational-age infants (Gillogley et al, 1990; Bingol et al, 1987; Chouteau et al, 1988; Little et al, 1989; Zuckerman et al, 1989; Fulroth et al, 1989) and this may be mediated through its appetite-suppressing effect (Riley, 1987) which also causes poor maternal weight gain.

Maternal effects

Maternal blood pressure and uterine vascular resistance are both increased while uterine blood flow is decreased by the use of cocaine (Woods et al, 1987). This response appears to be enhanced in pregnancy, possibly mediated by progesterone (Woods and Plessinger, 1990).

The incidence of arterial thromboses is also increased and this may be due to the reduced levels of protein C and antithrombin III found in these women (Choksi et al, 1989).

Maternal deaths have been reported due to:

- cardiac arrhythmias
- coronary ischaemia
- ruptured intracranial aneurysms
- intracerebral haemorrhage
- convulsions from raised blood pressure.

Fetal effects

Both the spontaneous and induced abortion rates are increased by cocaine addiction (Chasnoff et al, 1985; Gillogley et al, 1990). The incidence of abruption is reported to be raised and the stillbirth rate from abruption is increased tenfold (Bingol et al, 1987), possibly due to damage to placental/uterine vessels early in pregnancy.

Animal studies report numerous different malformations and there have been similar reports from human studies (Mahalik et al, 1980, 1984). However, others report no increase in the incidence of congenital anomalies (Gillogley et al, 1990; Fantel and MacPhail, 1982; Church et al, 1988). It is thought that the induced structural defects are not limited to the period of organogenesis but extend further in to fetal life. Alteration or reduction in uterine and hence placental and fetal blood flow in the second trimester may cause vascular disruptions such as intestinal atresia, limb reduction defects and genitourinary defects (Hoyme et al, 1990).

Intrauterine growth retardation (IUGR) is the most consistent finding in all studies. It is interesting to note that, unlike IUGR caused by opiate addiction, there does not appear to be 'head sparing'; that is, brain growth is impaired as well (Little and Snell, 1991; Zuckerman et al, 1989). Fat stores are reduced as is lean body mass and this may be due to impairment of nutrient transfer (Frank et al, 1990). If cocaine use is stopped before delivery, there may be some resumption of growth. However, neurobehavioural defects may still persist (Chasnoff et al, 1989).

The incidence of prematurity is increased (Gillogley et al, 1990; Little et al, 1989) but this is less clear than with opiates.

Neonatal effects

There is some debate as to whether this actually exists. If it does, the symptoms are:

- hypertonia
- hyperactive startle reflex
- tachypnoea
- loose stools
- reduced sleep (Fulroth et al, 1989).

One interesting finding is that if the woman uses cocaine as well as opiates, the NAS associated with opiate abuse is less severe (Finnegan et al, 1990).

Benzodiazepenes

Benzodiazepenes are one of the most commonly prescribed drugs in Britain and are very easily obtainable, especially temazepam. The effects of these drugs on pregnancy are uncertain but the use of diazepam in early pregnancy has been associated with an increased incidence of cleft palate, and doses of more than 30mg per day may result in neonatal withdrawal (Harrison, 1986), the symptoms being:

- hypotonia
- hypothermia
- hyperbilirubinaemia
- feeding difficulties with poor sucking
- respiratory difficulties with episodes of apnoea.

As mentioned above, the concomitant use of benzodiazepenes and opiates causes delay in the onset of neonatal abstinence syndrome associated with opiate abuse in pregnancy.

Amphetamines

Amphetamines are sympathomimetic drugs and are used most commonly for weight loss, since they are appetite suppressants, and for the treatment of narcolepsy as they are central nervous system (CNS) stimulants. Their use in pregnancy is not uncommon, often in association with other drugs.

There is little evidence regarding either specific or nonspecific effects in pregnancy. They do not appear to cause fetal anomalies but may be associated with an increase in small-for-gestational-age and preterm infants (Oro and Dixon, 1987).

Specific maternal effects which are not confined to pregnancy are hypertension, tachycardia and hyperthermia and thus the incidence of cerebrovascular accidents, myocardial infarction and cardiac arrhythmias may be increased in those with underlying pathology.

Marijuana

The effect of marijuana is uncertain. It is used most commonly together with tobacco and alcohol and thus it is difficult to identify effects specific to this drug.

Organization of care

Drug abusers can be identified among women attending for antenatal care by screening urine samples for drug metabolites. However, this is time consuming and may not be cost effective except perhaps in those areas where the incidence of drug abuse is particularly high. Ethically, without express consent, this sort of screening is highly dubious practice.

We are more likely to succeed in our aims, and the women are more likely to cooperate, if a 'team approach' is used, providing a comprehensive range of services including medical, social, psychological and psychiatric help with confidentiality guaranteed. This multidisciplinary approach should be maintained throughout pregnancy, delivery and the postpartum period not only for the woman but also for her infant and immediate family (Lief, 1985). Where possible, all drug-addicted pregnant patients should book under the care of an obstetric consultant within a unit who has declared a special interest in this problem. In addition, the involvement of a specially trained midwife will ensure continuity, and hopefully coordination, of care between hospital and community staff enabling those who fail to attend their hospital visits to be followed up outside of the hospital setting by someone familiar with their case/care. Registration of these women with the local drug unit will enable close monitoring of their drug-using habits during and after the pregnancy and provide an invaluable source of advice and support to both patient and professionals. Involvement of the GP is important, where the woman wishes it, and good channels of communication between consultant, GP, midwife and members of the drug unit staff should prevent confusion over management plans for individual patients.

Antenatal care

The aim of antenatal care for any pregnant woman is to ensure the safe delivery of a healthy mother and child. To ensure this for women who are drug users will require disproportionate input from all staff involved than would be necessary for the usually fit and healthy pregnant population.

Screening

In addition to the usual screening tests there are a number of other tests which may be indicated in this group. These women are prone to sexually-transmitted diseases (Strauss et al, 1974); thus they should be screened for the Hepatitis B surface antigen (HBSAg) and, where indicated, swabs may be taken for sexually-transmitted diseases. The question of screening for HIV is fraught with difficulties. Another important investigation is an ultrasound scan for gestational age. In units where it is not policy to perform this for all pregnant women, an exception should be made for drug users since their gestational age based on the last menstrual period is so unreliable. For those women who 'book late', parameters more accurate in late pregnancy, such as foot length and transcerebellar diameter, may be necessary.

Drug use

The aim should be to encourage a decrease or even total cessation of drug use. Where possible, transfer to legal alternatives is preferable to continued use of street drugs. At present this is only possible for heroin addicts where the legal alternative is methadone. Transfer on to this drug has many potential advantages.

The institution of a methadone maintenance programme brings the mother into contact with both medical and social support which may improve her standard of living sufficiently to benefit both the mother's and infant's health (Rosner et al, 1982). It ensures contact is maintained with medical services as this is necessary to obtain a regular supply of the drug. It should reduce the incidence of withdrawal because the supply is constant as it is taken at regular intervals and thus the normal peaks and troughs which occur with heroin use are abolished (Finnegan, 1991). This in turn should reduce the incidence of fetal withdrawal, meconium staining of liquor and intrauterine deaths (Strauss et al, 1974).

The dose of methadone will need adjusting during pregnancy. Initially conversion to methadone from heroin is needed if this has not already been done prior to pregnancy. This requires the experience and skill of those professionals who work in this field on a daily basis. Once stabilized on methadone, consideration can be given to reducing the dose. If this is to be done it should be done slowly at a rate of no more than 5mg reductions per week. Often it is possible to reduce the dose in the second trimester only to find that it needs increasing again later in pregnancy because of the altered pharmacokinetics of the drug caused by pregnancy physiology (Pond et al, 1985).

The disadvantage of maintenance on methadone is that it has a much longer half life than heroin so that not only are neonatal withdrawal symptoms more severe, they can also be delayed and last longer (Perlmutter, 1974; Blinick et al, 1976; Strauss et al, 1974). Unfortunately, there is no legal substitute for cocaine or any of the other drugs of abuse. The only option in these cases (when and if the women admit to their use) is to persuade them to reduce or cease their intake.

Drug use can be monitored during pregnancy, and at any other time, by testing urine for drug metabolites, with maternal consent.

Fetal monitoring

Fetal growth is a major concern in these women, the majority of whom not only use illicit drugs but also smoke tobacco which causes a dose-related reduction in birthweight (Kline et al, 1987). Regular antenatal checks are necessary and serial ultrasound measurements for growth are advisable. As with any other pregnant woman, advice should be given regarding fetal movements in the third trimester.

Labour and delivery

The fact that a woman is known to be a drug user should have little if any effect on her management during labour or afterwards, with a few exceptions.

Women who have used drugs intravenously are likely to have poor venous access which may cause problems if faced with an intrapartum emergency. Similarly adequate analgesia can be difficult to provide in both opiate and cocaine addicts especially if the analgesic chosen is an opiate. Much higher doses than normal may be required and even then may not be effective. Epidural analgesia is an alternative in those women who find this acceptable.

Intrapartum fetal monitoring may be difficult due to the effects of opiates on fetal heart rate patterns. There may be reduced baseline variability, loss of accelerations and, as mentioned above, intrapartum fetal withdrawal may result in unusual CTG patterns, all of which make interpretation of these cardiotocographs difficult.

Other complications of pregnancy described above will dictate management of specific cases during labour as with any other pregnancy. The management of HBSAg and HIV positive women should be as for any other woman so affected. Although drug users are more likely to be positive for these infections, management of any situation where contact with body fluids is likely should be one of great care, regardless of a person's admitted drug habits and should follow established guidelines.

Ongoing care

Pregnancy is a unique episode in a woman's life and, as such, should be 'exploited' as an opportunity to encourage change in the woman's lifestyle to eliminate habits which are potentially dangerous, not just for her baby, but also herself. The use of illicit drugs during pregnancy is, as can be seen, dangerous for both mother and child. The risk does not necessarily diminish after birth. The most important factor in long-term success in breaking an addictive habit is a change in lifestyle (Oppenheimer et al, 1979) and thus support after delivery from the appropriately qualified personnel is imperative.

About the authors

Dr Colette Sparey is currently a Registrar in Obstetrics and Gynaecology at the Liverpool Maternity and Women's Hospitals. She qualified in July 1987 at Manchester University and has worked primarily in obstetrics and gynaecology since then.

Mr Steve Walkinshaw is currently consultant in Maternal Fetal Medicine at the Liverpool Women's Hospital, which is one of only two Trusts solely devoted to the care of women. Clinically he is a trained subspecialist in Fetal Medicine and responsible for the provision of specialist care in Liverpool and the North West region. He was involved in the Joint Colleges forum on Changing Childbirth and on the NHS Executive Group discussing joint educational initiatives. As Clinical Director he was actively involved in the developing of the Changing Childbirth model for implementation within Liverpool. His clinical interests are prenatal diagnosis, intrapartum care and late pregnancy antenatal monitoring.

CHAPTER FIVE

Hepatitis B, Pregnancy and the Drug User

PETER CAREY

Hepatitis B virus (HBV) infection is present throughout the world and it has been estimated that there are 400–500 million people chronically infected: HBV carriers (Moradpour and Wands, 1995). Instrumental in maintaining high prevalence in certain developing countries are mother to baby transmission and horizontal transmission within families and between young people in schools. In many developed countries HBV is mainly transmitted between adults. In the UK it has been estimated that 0.1 per cent of the population are HBV carriers. Drug users may be at risk of HBV infection if they inject drugs and share their injecting equipment. Drugs cost money and some users may have to work in the sex industry in order to pay for their drugs or exchange sex for drugs, thus putting themselves at risk potentially of HBV and other sexually transmissible infections. A pregnant HBV infected drug user may transmit HBV to her baby.

The virus

HBV is an enveloped DNA virus with three major antigenic determinants.

1. Hepatitis B surface antigen : HBsAg
2. Hepatitis B core antigen : HBcAg
3. Hepatitis B e antigen : HBeAg

HBsAg is found in the surface envelope whilst HBcAg and HBeAg are found in the viral core together with viral DNA and DNA polymerase required for viral replication within infected hepatocytes.

Infected individuals will have HBV in a variety of body fluids including blood, seminal fluid, vaginal fluid and saliva. The incubation period for hepatitis B is usually within three months of infection. Many infections are asymptomatic, particularly in children. Complete recovery characterizes most acute infections. Fulminant HBV infection is rare and may be associated with HBV mutations lacking HBeAg.

A small proportion of infected adults fail to clear HBV, remain infected and become carriers. An HBV carrier is defined as someone who remains HBsAg positive for more than six months following infection. A proportion of these people will eventually develop chronic hepatitis, cirrhosis or hepatocellular carcinoma. Generally speaking HBV transmission may occur in one of four ways.

1. Parenteral
2. Sexual
3. Mother to Baby
4. Horizontal

Screening of blood donors has dramatically reduced HBV infection associated with blood transfusion although parenteral spread of HBV remains common amongst injecting drug users (IDUs) who share their injecting equipment. Parenteral infection of health care workers (HCWs), for instance as a result of needle-stick injury, is largely preventable as a result of HBV vaccination programs, although a small proportion of vaccinees fail to respond. Proper attention to infection control and needle-stick injury policies and correct disposal of sharp instruments is mandatory!

Sexual transmission of HBV may occur as a result of vaginal or anal intercourse with an infected partner.

Horizontal transmission of HBV from an HBV carrier to family members may occur and is a likely method of transmission to children in countries with high endemicity for the virus. Uncertainty surrounds the mechanism for such transmissions but may be associated with accidental parenteral exposure to blood or saliva or with mouth to mouth transmission.

Mother to baby transmission

Acute HBV infection during the second half of pregnancy, particularly during the third trimester, may lead to intrauterine infection. HBV carrier mothers may infect their babies intrapartum either from micro-transfusion of blood or from direct contact with HBV infected blood or mucus. Breastfeeding is not thought to be important in mother to baby transmission (Vajro and Fontanella, 1991), but it has been suggested that transmission may occur from HBV infected mothers who masticate their babies' food.

Diagnosis

During acute infection HBsAg is usually the first serological marker to become positive, followed by HBeAg and then the antibodies: antiHBc IgM and anti HBc IgG to core antigen; anti HBe to e antigen; and anti HBs to surface antigen.

In those who recover from infection HBeAg disappears after several weeks associated with the appearance of anti HBe. HBsAg disappears later followed eventually by the appearance of anti HBs with the persistence of anti HBc IgG.

Chronic HBV infection is associated with the persistence of HBsAg (a proportion of individuals will also have HBeAg) and HBc IgG. The degree of altered liver function as shown by increased alanine aminotransferase (ALT) in the diagram below varies according to the severity of hepatitis (taken from C.G. Teo. 'The virology and serology of hepatitis: an overview.' *Communicable Diseases Report*, 1992; 2: R109–14).

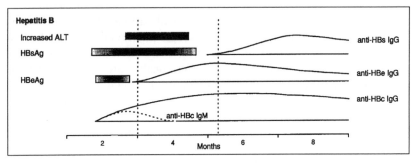

Fig. 5.1: The chronology of infection with hepatitis B

The presence of HBeAg in the blood of an HBV carrier is associated with high infectivity increasing the likelihood of HBV transmission irrespective of the mode of transmission. Loss of HBeAg with seroconversion to anti HBe is associated with lower infectivity.

Maternal disease

HBV infection in adults is usually associated with clearing of virus and lifelong immunity but about 5–10 per cent become carriers. In our local maternity hospital most pregnant drug users with HBV infection are carriers.

The course of HBV infection in pregnancy is said to be no different to that in non-pregnant women. In those developing icteric disease the period of jaundice is usually limited to about four weeks and may be presaged in the preceding week by a prodrome resembling serum sickness, due to the circulation of immune complexes. Urticaria, arthralgia or arthropathy may develop. The syndrome may be seen also in people without jaundice.

In most cases women can be managed at home unless complicating factors supervene such as recurrent vomiting, anorexia or fulminant hepatitis. Periods of rest should be encouraged with avoidance of prolonged or excessive physical activity. There are no specific dietary restrictions but individuals are advised against alcoholic drinks as they may exacerbate liver dysfunction. All unnecessary drugs should be stopped. Such advice given to drug users may lead to serious withdrawal symptoms if taken literally and management should be coordinated with the drug liaison midwife and the local Drug Dependency Clinic with respect to continuing drug use, such as methadone maintenance.

The most serious complication of HBV infection in pregnancy is the development of fulminant hepatitis which may progress rapidly to hepatic failure and death in 70–95 per cent of patients. Bleeding problems may develop secondary to impaired production of coagulation factors, whilst respiratory distress syndrome or sepsis may be added complications.

There is no specific treatment for fulminant hepatitis other than intensive support, correction of coagulopathy and proper management of other complications such as sepsis. The risk of fulminant hepatitis is said to be less than two per cent.

Management by experienced specialists in the Intensive Care Unit provides the best environment for monitoring and intervention. Liver transplantation has been suggested for women in whom recovery from hepatitis is unlikely. No convincing data exist as to whether caesarean section, induction of labour or termination of pregnancy are of benefit to mother or fetus. For a more complete account of hepatitis B infection the reader should consult standard texts.

Effect of HBV on pregnancy outcome

Premature delivery (before gestational age of 37 weeks) is said to be two to three times more common in pregnant women with hepatitis, irrespective of the causal virus, compared with non-infected pregnant women and is most likely to occur associated with hepatitis in the third trimester.

Fulminant hepatitis in pregnancy leads to fetal death in about 70 per cent of cases but is not a feature of uncomplicated HBV infection.

Consequences for baby

Mothers with HBV infection who are HBeAg positive have about an 85 per cent chance of infecting their babies compared with a 31 per cent chance if they are HBeAg negative (Beasley et al, 1977). Chronic HBV infection will develop in about 90 per cent of these babies, most of whom will have experienced asymptomatic infection although severe hepatitis will be seen in a small proportion.

Most babies who acquire HBV infection from their mothers do so during delivery and so serological tests for infection will be negative initially, seroconversion occurring during the first three months of life.

HBV infection persists for many years as shown by HBeAg and/or HBsAg positivity. Chronic active hepatitis or hepatocellular carcinoma may be long-term sequelae.

Prevention of mother to baby transmission

In the UK hepatitis B immunisation is not included in recommended immunisation schedules. Methods to reduce the prevalence of HBV in the population such as screening blood donors, heat treating blood products, education about safer sex, specific advice to IDUs and their partners and the availability of syringe schemes will all help to reduce HBV infection in pregnant women, including the pregnant drug user. Identifying those at risk of HBV infection and immunising susceptible individuals is the strategy adopted in this country in the absence of routine immunisation of children or adolescents.

The vaccine contains HBsAg prepared from yeast cells using recombinant DNA techniques. 1ml of vaccine contains 20micrograms of HBsAg. Vaccine should be stored between 2° and 8°C. Freezing destroys the vaccine's potency. (Manufacturers recommendations, Engerix B, SmithKline Beecham Pharmaceuticals.)

Immunisation stimulates the production of antibodies (anti HBs) against HBsAg and levels exceeding 100 IU/L are considered to be protective. Over 90 per cent of immunised individuals respond satisfactorily. Poor response to immunisation may be associated with HIV infection, other types of immunosuppression, presence of HLA B8 haplotype, age over 50, incorrect immunisation technique, e.g. injection of vaccine into the buttock, or inactivation of vaccine (see above).

Antibody levels should be checked about two months after completion of immunisation and if between 10–100 IU/L (poor responders) or less than 10 IU/L (non responders) a booster dose should be offered with further assessment of anti HBs. If response remains poor reimmunisation should be considered. Double doses of vaccine may be required for some people though such use is outside the product license.

Protective antibody levels remain for variable periods of time in different individuals and may be predicted from initial response to immunisation. Booster immunisation for good responders is recommended at between three and five years following initial immunisation, for those who require continuing protection against HBV infection.

Procedure

Active immunisation is commenced by the intramuscular injection of 1ml of hepatitis B vaccine into the deltoid muscle. This is repeated at one month and again at six months following the initial dose. Alternatively an accelerated course may be used for more rapid immunisation. Following the initial dose of vaccine repeat doses are given at one and two months followed by a booster at 12 months. This may be used for those requiring more rapid protection such as travellers abroad or for those exposed parenterally or sexually to HBV, when this active immunisation is combined with passive immunisation with hepatitis B immunoglobulin (HBIG).

Immunisation is usually well tolerated. The most common side-effect is pain at the injection site, though fever, rash, malaise and flu-like symptoms have been reported.

The presence of severe febrile infection is considered to be a reason for postponing immunisation.

Susceptible pregnant drug users at risk of HBV infection should be offered active immunisation.

Passive immunisation with HBIG is available for susceptible people exposed parenterally or sexually to HBV. In the UK small stocks of HBIG are held by the Public Health Laboratory Services who will also give advice about the procedure. 500 IU is given by intramuscular injection whilst commencing active immunisation at a different site. The accelerated course may be used. It is advisable to immunise within 48 hours of parenteral exposure and within 14 days following sexual exposure, the sooner the better.

Some mothers will be identified as having HBV infection during pregnancy. Protection of their infants involves passive immunisation with HBIG by intramuscular injection into the anterolateral aspect of the baby's thigh within 12 hours and certainly no later than 48 hours after birth. Ten micrograms of hepatitis B vaccine is given into the opposite thigh at the same time followed by repeat doses at one and six months. About 95 per cent of babies will be protected against HBV infection in this way. HBV serology should be assessed at 12 months of age. Further information with respect to active and passive immunisation against HBV infection may be found in the HMSO publication *Immunisation against Infectious Diseases* (HMSO, 1992).

After delivery mother and baby may remain together if their clinical status allows. Although HBV has been found in breastmilk there are no data to suggest that breastfeeding carries an increased risk of transmission and so breastfeeding is allowed if mother wishes this. Proper infection control in the delivery suite should be observed and mother advised about good hygiene and how to deal with lochia. Whilst protection against HBV is well established no immunisation schedule is available to protect against hepatitis C virus (HCV). This RNA virus is transmitted principally in blood but sexual and mother to baby transmission have been described. Infection is usually inapparent but can lead to chronic liver disease in up to 50 per cent of people. Diagnosis is made on the basis of finding antibodies to HCV, anti HCV IgG, in the serum of infected people. Mother to baby spread seems to be associated with viraemia detected by the presence of high titred HCV RNA using PCR (Alter, 1994). Coinfection with HIV seems to be a risk factor for this route of transmission (Zanetti et al, 1995). Blood/organ donors are routinely screened for HCV infection.

Hepatitis D virus (HDV or delta agent) is an incomplete RNA virus which becomes enveloped by HBsAg in order to establish infection (see diagram below taken from Teo, 1992, *op. cit.*). Characteristically transmitted in blood, sexual spread is also possible. Individuals may be coinfected with HBV and HDV or HBV carriers may be superinfected with HDV. The latter situation may lead to severe hepatitis with progression to chronic liver disease. Serological tests for HDV are available.

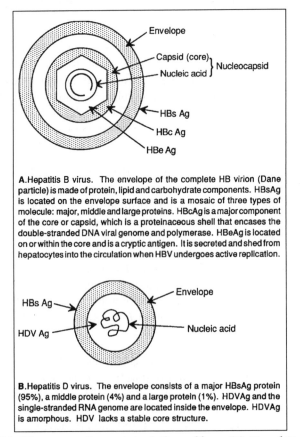

A.Hepatitis B virus. The envelope of the complete HB virion (Dane particle) is made of protein, lipid and carbohydrate components. HBsAg is located on the envelope surface and is a mosaic of three types of molecule: major, middle and large proteins. HBcAg is a major component of the core or capsid, which is a proteinaceous shell that encases the double-stranded DNA viral genome and polymerase. HBeAg is located on or within the core and is a cryptic antigen. It is secreted and shed from hepatocytes into the circulation when HBV undergoes active replication.

B.Hepatitis D virus. The envelope consists of a major HBsAg protein (95%), a middle protein (4%) and a large protein (1%). HDVAg and the single-stranded RNA genome are located inside the envelope. HDVAg is amorphous. HDV lacks a stable core structure.

Fig. 5.2: Diagrammatic representation of hepatitis B and D viruses

Immunisation against HBV will protect against HDV infection but HBV carriers cannot be immunised against HDV and thus remain at risk of infection from this virus and indeed HCV as well, if they continue risky practices such as sharing drug injecting equipment.

Individuals who have chronic HBV infection should be counselled about the possibility of other household members or sexual partner(s) being at risk from infection and HBV screening offered to those willing to be tested. Those who are susceptible can be identified and offered HBV vaccination.

Concluding remarks

Much can be done to prevent the spread of HBV in the community. It is better to prevent HBV infection than to manage it in the pregnant drug user. Once identified however, mother to baby transmission can be prevented in most cases. Mothers with chronic HBV infection should be referred for specialist assessment following the completion of pregnancy. Some may benefit from therapy with interferon alpha as may some with chronic HCV infection.

Users who continue to inject should be strongly advised about harm minimization, in particular about the use of sterile equipment and not sharing injecting equipment with others. The topic is dealt with elsewhere in this book. This will protect against blood borne viruses such as HBV, HCV, HDV and human immunodeficiency virus (HIV) and infections with bacteria or yeasts which may be introduced into the body by the use of unsterile equipment.

Safer sex practices (see chapter on sexually transmitted diseases) should also be discussed particularly for users whose income for purchase of drugs relies on work in the sex industry or exchange of sexual favours for drugs.

About the author

Dr Peter Carey qualified at Liverpool University in 1970. He is a Fellow of the Royal College of Physicians and has been a consultant in Genitourinary Medicine in Liverpool for 16 years. He has developed a specialist interest in HIV medicine during the last 11 years. He has outpatient and inpatient responsibilities in the Royal Liverpool and Broadgreen University Hospital NHS Trust together with a contribution to community care. He is an honorary lecturer at Liverpool University.

CHAPTER SIX

Human Immunodeficiency Virus, Pregnancy and the Drug User

PETER CAREY

Introduction

Since the first descriptions of Acquired Immune Deficiency Syndrome (AIDS) in 1981, AIDS has become pandemic having been reported from 192 countries throughout the world.

Africa	347,713
Americas	526,682
Asia	17,057
Europe	127,886
Oceania	5,735
Total	**1,025,073**

(from *Weekly Epidemiological Record*, No. 2, Jan. 1995)

The World Health Organization (WHO) estimates that over 16 million adults and more than one million children have been infected so far.

HIV, the cause of AIDS was discovered in 1983 and renamed HIV-1 in 1986 following the identification of an HIV variant: HIV-2 in West Africa. HIV-1 is the predominant virus throughout the world and at least five different sub-types have been identified. HIV-2 is less easily transmitted than HIV-1, either sexually or from mother to baby and seems to produce slower disease progression to AIDS (O'Shaughnessy and Schechter, 1994).

HIV may be transmitted either sexually, via infected blood or blood products or from mother to baby.

The epidemiology of HIV infection is complex varying from country to country and within countries. Sexual transmission of HIV between men and women is the most commonly associated risk factor in many countries whilst sex between men or sharing of drug injecting equipment are important in others.

HIV infection associated with the transfusion of blood or blood products has been reduced dramatically in most countries because of screening of blood donors and heat treatment of factor VIII. HIV transmission from transfused blood may still be a problem in those parts of the world where screening of all blood donors cannot be accomplished, and nosocomial transmission of HIV has been described from the reuse of needles and syringes.

In the UK the cumulative total for people with HIV-1 infection is 23,934 (including 10,693 people with AIDS). 3,391 women with HIV-1 infection have been reported including 844 who are injecting drug users (IDUs). Seven hundred and nineteen babies have been born to mothers with HIV-1 infection. Of these 290 were HIV infected and 234 escaped infection; 205 were of undetermined status and continuing follow-up (*Communicable Diseases Report*, 1995).

In the absence of an effective vaccine or 'cure', recognition of the ways in which HIV is transmitted allows for the development of appropriate strategies to prevent the spread of the virus. Screening of blood/organ donors and heat treatment of factor VIII are now well established ways of protecting recipients from infection. Education for sexually active people (and indeed before they become sexually active) about safer sex and harm minimization for IDUs are similarly crucial in reducing the spread of HIV in communities. Programmes to control the spread of sexually transmitted diseases (STDs) will per se control the sexual spread of HIV. Some STDs, for instance those causing genital ulcer disease, may be cofactors for the acquisition of HIV, further emphasizing the importance of disease control.

HIV in pregnancy

The diagnosis of HIV infection in pregnancy causes much anxiety for women, their partners and their families, although some women who are aware of their HIV status choose to become pregnant. Many questions may be asked:

*   Should I continue with my pregnancy?
*   What are the chances of my baby being infected?
*   If my baby is infected will he or she develop AIDS?
*   Will pregnancy make my HIV infection worse?
*   Who will look after my baby if I die?
*   Does my partner have HIV infection?
*   Are any of my children infected?
*   Who should I tell?

These and other questions demand time and consideration to answer. Some women may choose to continue with their pregnancies whilst others will request termination. In either situation counselling and long-term support will be required. The midwife would seem to be in an ideal position to give help, provided that she has the knowledge and skills.

For the pregnant drug user who has HIV infection there is the added worry of the effect of her drug use on the fetus and pregnancy outcome. The remainder of this chapter attempts to deal with these problems.

HIV testing

Many centres now offer a same day testing service where, following appropriate counselling, blood is drawn for an HIV test in the morning with a result available later in the afternoon. The timing of the test with respect to potential exposure is important, remembering that after HIV infection, seroconversion may take up to three months and occasionally longer. Positive results must be double checked against a further blood sample from the individual concerned. The necessary support services should be available to provide comprehensive assistance as and when required. This may require expertise from a specialist centre if not available within the maternity unit. Centres which regularly offer HIV testing include Drug Dependency Clinics, Genitourinary Medicine Departments, Infectious Diseases Units and Syringe Exchange Schemes.

HIV testing may be requested for other family members and should be undertaken with similar expedition and sensitivity remembering that such testing remains a voluntary activity and individuals are not consenting to be tested for the doctor's benefit. HIV infection is not just a problem for the individual; it becomes a problem for the family as well if they are chosen to be involved, thus support should extend to those family members who require it.

The care of an HIV infected drug user during pregnancy demands the close cooperation of the obstetric team (Obstetrician, Midwife, Drug Liaison Midwife) the Drug Dependency Clinic and Specialist in HIV medicine.

The monitoring of fetal development at appropriate intervals should be linked with close monitoring of drug use and education around harm minimization. Regular medical supervision of HIV disease is also necessary with additional support from the counselling team.

The effect of pregnancy on HIV disease

During 'normal' pregnancy CD4 + lymphocytes (T4 helper cells) decline to a nadir during the third trimester recovering to pre-pregnancy levels at about term (Tallon et al, 1984). CD4 + lymphocyte function seems to be normal as does B cell function. Mildly depressed cell mediated immunity does occur, however, and may be associated with increased levels of circulating hormones. This may be associated with increased severity of certain infections in some women such as genital warts or malaria.

HIV infection in pregnancy seems to be associated with a more rapid fall in CD4 + lymphocytes but without recovery to pre-pregnancy levels at term (Biggar et al, 1989). Furthermore it has been suggested that the use of illicit drugs in pregnancy may be associated with CD4 + lymphocyte decline.

When CD4 + lymphocytes fall below 0.2 x 10^9/L (200/ml of blood) prophylaxis begins to prevent pneumocystis carinii pneumonia (PCP); a most important AIDS defining illness. Although the natural history of HIV infection both during and after pregnancy needs to be more clearly defined, it is felt generally that pregnancy does not affect HIV disease progression in the asymptomatic woman. However, earlier research suggested that AIDS in pregnancy might reduce survival. PCP was the leading cause of death in one retrospective study. PCP prophylaxis should considerably reduce this problem whilst correct management of acute PCP should improve survival. More recent research has suggested that survival time was not reduced in AIDS related pregnancies.

Medical care

Regular health checks, often driven by the mother's own needs, are advised during the course of pregnancy allowing for symptomatic review and clinical examination. Visits tend to be more frequent in women with symptomatic disease. Most women will be offered a screen for STDs including syphilis, hepatitis B and also hepatitis C. New genital symptoms, genital symptoms in a sexual partner or casual unprotected sexual intercourse would be reasons for offering repeat tests and reinforcing advice about safer sexual practices.

Full blood count, liver and renal function tests, viral studies and urinalysis are included in the standard investigations whilst CD4 + lymphocyte levels are monitored throughout pregnancy. Primary PCP prophylaxis is recommended when counts fall below 200/ml; co-trimoxazole 960mg on alternate days being the treatment of choice.

Problems such as oral candidosis and fungal infections of skin are usually easily managed with the prescription of topical anti-fungal agents but in-patient care in a specialist unit is required if opportunistic infections develop. For instance PCP requires treatment with high dose intravenous co-trimoxazole combined with corticosteroids in the presence of respiratory failure, together with appropriate administration of oxygen. Secondary prophylaxis with co-trimoxazole follows acute treatment to prevent recurrence.

Other opportunistic infections should be managed appropriately with the recognition that some commonly used drugs may have the potential for fetal damage. Fortunately Karposi's sarcoma, an important AIDS defining tumour, is uncommon in IDUs and in women.

Drug users who continue to inject during pregnancy may have problems related to these activities. Infection problems such as skin abscess, cellulitis, septicaemia, pnuemonia or endocarditis may occur. Tuberculosis is found more commonly in IDUs than in the population in general, being a particular problem in New York City. It is less commonly found in IDUs in the UK. These issues are dealt with elsewhere in this book. The immunosupression associated with HIV infection could exacerbate these complications and management in a specialist unit is mandatory.

Symptoms secondary to drug use may mimic those associated with HIV related problems, for instance drug users withdrawing from benzodiazapines may experience seizures as may HIV infected individuals who have cerebral toxoplasmosis or lymphoma. The caring team needs to be well aware of these problems. Two excellent reviews are referenced at the end of this book (Selwyn and O'Connor, 1992; Sherrard, Bingham and Owen, 1993). Issues around zidovudine prescription are dealt with later.

Effect of HIV on pregnancy and fetus

Research from New York and Edinburgh suggested that women with HIV associated pregnancies were no more likely than HIV negative controls to choose termination of pregnancy.

A study of pregnant IDUs with HIV infection in New York showed no association between HIV infection, spontaneous abortion, preterm delivery, still birth or low birthweight, compared with non-HIV infected IDUs. Other studies have confirmed these results. Conversely African studies in non-IDU pregnancies note a variety of pregnancy complications such as preterm labour and low birthweight, but general agreement about the association of low birthweight and HIV infection. In these studies there is some suggestion that low birthweight may be related to the stage of maternal infection in pregnancy.

Congenital abnormalities do not seem to be found more commonly in HIV-related pregnancies and initial reports suggesting a specific dysmorphic syndrome have not been confirmed.

Mother to baby transmission

Research has suggested that the fetus can be infected as early as the first or second trimesters and that intrapartum infection of the baby is also significant. The relative importance of each awaits clarification.

Primary infection during pregnancy may be a risk factor for some because of the associated rapid viral replication and high viral load. Similarly in symptomatic mothers with advancing disease the risk of HIV transmission seems to increase. This is usually associated with low CD4 + lymphocyte counts and raised p24 antigen levels associated with increased viral load. Lack of neutralizing antibodies to HIV may also be a factor whilst some HIV strains may be more able inherently to infect the fetus or baby. Certain STDs such as those associated with genital ulcers may also be risk factors for transmission as may be the presence of chorioamnionitis at term.

Mode of delivery may play some part in mother to baby transmission with studies showing some protection from caesarean section compared with vaginal delivery. Premature rupture of membranes and prolonged labour are likely to increase exposure to maternal virus.

Various studies show that the risk of mother to baby transmission of HIV ranges from 14–39 per cent with the lowest estimate coming from the European Collaborative Study (Newell, Dunn and Peckham, 1992).

Transmission during breastfeeding was first described in mothers postnatally infected with HIV. Estimates suggest that women postnatally infected with HIV have a 29 per cent chance of transmitting infection during breastfeeding. Subsequent research suggests an additional 14 per cent risk of transmission for mothers with established HIV infection who breastfed their babies following vaginal delivery.

Factors involving transmission as a result of breastfeeding have been studied and suggest that virally infected cells in breastmilk may be important while persistence of HIV IgM antibodies in breastmilk may be associated with decreased transmission. Substances that inhibit binding of HIV to CD4 + cells have also been found in breastmilk.

Prevention of transmission

Intrauterine HIV infection of the fetus may occur via the transplacental route whilst infection during delivery may be consequent upon:

1. materno-fetal transfusion of HIV infected blood;
2. direct exposure to HIV infected blood during delivery;
3. exposure to HIV present in cervical mucus or vaginal fluid.

A study published recently showed the effect of zidovudine in reducing mother to baby transmission in HIV-1 infection (Connor et al, 1994). HIV infected mothers in the second or third trimesters were randomized to receive zidovudine or placebo with a resulting two-thirds reduction of transmission in the zidovudine group. Treated mothers were given intravenous zidovudine during labour and their babies given zidovudine suspension during their first six weeks of life. Mothers were minimally symptomatic with CD4 + lymphocyte counts greater than 200/ml and had not taken zidovudine previously. Mothers seemed to tolerate the drug well.

Zidovudine crosses the placenta and has so far not been associated with fetal malformations but babies in the zidovudine group had lower haemoglobins than those in the placebo group. The long-term consequences of fetal exposure to zidovudine are not known and the mechanism for reducing transmission is not clear. The study had three arms; antepartum, intrapartum and postpartum. It is not known whether one or more of these interventions is instrumental in reducing mother to baby transmission. Will zidovudine be of benefit to symptomatic mothers with more advanced disease or to those who have taken zidovudine previously?

This study has thrown up many questions and its results should be discussed carefully with individuals who might benefit potentially from such prescription.

A meta-analysis of several prospective studies suggested that caesarean section reduced transmission of HIV by 30 per cent whilst work from the European Collaborative Study suggested that caesarean section halved mother to baby transmission (European Collaborative Study, 1993). Whether these studies will modify clinical practice in the future remains to be seen but it may be very difficult to randomize pregnant mothers into caesarean or vaginal delivery groups to answer this question satisfactorily.

Finally vaginal cleansing procedures are being researched in an effort to reduce exposure of baby to maternal HIV during birth. Povidone iodine and chlorhexidine have been assessed.

Whatever the mode of delivery proper infection control procedures should be observed by maternity staff and following delivery mothers should be advised about good hygiene and how to deal with lochia.

In the UK HIV infected mothers are advised not to breastfeed their babies, bottle feeding with appropriate formula feeds being substituted. However in parts of the world where this cannot be satisfactorily organized and where breastfeeding is important in providing babies with specific immunity against certain infectious diseases, advice not to breastfeed could be disastrous.

Follow-up of mother: postpartum

Regular health checks with respect to HIV infection should continue and these should include cervical cytology as women with HIV infection seem to have a greater likelihood of developing cervical intraepithelial neoplasia compared with HIV negative women.

Advice about safer sex should be offered again emphasizing the success of condom use. The European Study Group showed no seroconversion for HIV amongst 124 couples using condoms consistently during 15,000 episodes of sexual intercourse (De Vincenzi, 1994). Appropriate contraception should also be discussed. Insertion of IUCD is not recommended.

If mother has symptomatic HIV disease she may require help with her baby at home and this may be arranged via her family doctor or through local support agencies.

Follow-up of baby

Historically the diagnosis of HIV infection in babies has demanded follow-up for a minimum of 18 months to allow for the disappearance of passively transferred maternal antibody. Those with HIV serpositivity after this time are infected with HIV. In those babies not infected 50 per cent will be seronegative by ten months of life. Some babies will develop AIDS defining illnesses during this 18 months follow-up.

Some centres are able to culture HIV from babies lymphocytes or to look for the genetic material of HIV using polymerase chain reaction (PCR). Both are sensitive in the diagnosis of HIV infection after the age of two months. The development of assays to measure antibodies produced specifically by HIV-infected babies should also be useful in earlier detection of infection, for example IgA antibodies to HIV.

It has been estimated by the European Collaborative Group that 23 per cent of infected babies develop AIDS within the first year of life with a death rate of ten per cent, 40 per cent of children develop AIDS within four years and that 75 per cent of HIV-infected children are alive aged five years (Newell, 1993). The Italian HIV registry shows 70 per cent survival at six years and 50 per cent survival at nine years for HIV infected children (Tovo et al, 1992).

The management of babies born to mothers with HIV infection is beyond the scope of this chapter but care should be undertaken where possible with a specialist unit skilled in the management of such problems. Usual vaccination schedules are followed with the substitution of killed polio vaccine for the live attenuated form (HMSO, 1992). Careful consideration must be given to PCP prophylaxis.

Considerable family support may be required if the baby has HIV infection. Such a diagnosis may remain, sadly, both stigmatizing and isolating for many. Mother may feel guilty about 'infecting her child' and skilled counselling and support should be available for her. Careful supervision of drug use during this time is essential lest anxiety or depression from these events stimulate chaotic drug use.

About the author

Dr Peter Carey qualified at Liverpool University in 1970. He is a Fellow of the Royal College of Physicians and has been a consultant in Genitourinary Medicine in Liverpool for 16 years. He has developed a specialist interest in HIV medicine during the last 11 years. He has outpatient and inpatient responsibilities in the Royal Liverpool and Broadgreen University Hospital NHS Trust together with a contribution to community care. He is an honorary lecturer at Liverpool University.

CHAPTER SEVEN

The Sexual Health Needs of Female Drug Users

CLIVE L. MORRISON

Drug users as a group poorly utilize traditional health care services and female drug users in particular attend family planning clinics infrequently. Less than a tenth of drug-using prostitutes in Liverpool had ever attended a Genito-Urinary Medicine (GUM) service in the previous 12 months.

This means that these women do not have accurate information on sexual health, contraception or sexually transmitted diseases (STDs). Drug services tend to concentrate their HIV prevention strategy on the reduction of injection equipment-sharing, although most HIV infection is acquired sexually. Changing sharing behaviour has been a lot easier to achieve with the provision of Needle and Syringe Exchanges (NSE) than changing sexual risk behaviour in drug users through safer sex promotion.

Most female drug users are sexually active (84 per cent). Nearly a third will have an injecting, drug-using male partner. Although drug-using prostitutes usually claim to use safer sex techniques and condoms with their clients, less than a sixth will use condoms with their regular partner and only a quarter of all female drug users use any form of contraception.

There is always much discussion in the research literature of the uninhibiting effects of drug use during sexual activity and users being less likely to use safer sex and condoms. A significant proportion of prostitutes may use drugs while working for a variety of reasons but this is practically never a problem in the general population of female users.

Studies in the United States have made an Association between drug use (especially cocaine) and STDs and syphilis. Over 58 per cent of prostitutes in Liverpool use cocaine and there has been no evidence of syphilis or other STDs in those screened in the Maryland Centre. This is probably more a reflection on the poor delivery of HIV and STD prevention services in the US, particularly via outreach.

Why drug-using women infrequently use condoms is difficult to assess. Over half of those using condoms are dissatisfied with their use. A quarter of opiate-dependent women experience amenorrhoea and often believe that they cannot become pregnant. The levels of knowledge concerning fertility may be low, as sex education at school may not have been available to them. Some women may be in a relationship where they are not empowered enough or have insufficient negotiating skills to encourage a dominating male partner to use condoms. Cultural and religious beliefs will also have an influence. Apart from prostitutes, female drug users have infrequent partner change and may perceive monogamous relationships as having no risk. If the traditional services fail the female drug user, then the onus is on drug workers to provide the advice and information that is required to reduce the risks of sexual behaviour. Unfortunately drug workers have not addressed these issues sufficiently well enough recently as sexual health and drug misuse were fields apart until the advent of HIV.

Drugs and sexual health

The misuse of opiates can suppress the production of luteinizing hormone and follicle-stimulating hormone from the pituitary gland. This disturbance in hormonal balance prevents menstruation but this does not necessarily prevent fertility or ovulation. Heavy opiate use may cause additional amenorrhoea by a different mechanism. Opiate use and a chaotic lifestyle suppresses appetite with a consequent nutritional deficiency. Associated with weight loss is the cessation of menstruation.

Women commencing methadone programmes have found that their periods return within a short period of time and become pregnant unexpectedly as they still think their fertility is suppressed. Contraceptive advice and/or prescriptions should be given to women when they commence such programmes.

Use of other drugs such as amphetamines, cocaine and the psychedelic drugs have not been shown to interfere with the female reproductive system. There is also no interaction between any of the illicit drugs and the available forms of contraception which reduces their effectiveness nor any research to suggest that the side effects are increased.

Some women have reported that whilst using stimulant drugs they do not produce sufficient vaginal lubrication during sexual intercourse and this may cause internal injury. It is recommended that they use a lubricant such as KY Jelly.

The contraceptives

Barrier methods

The HIV virus cannot pass through a condom. However, condom failure is reported and this is generally as a result of poor technique. Condoms can split during sexual intercourse or come off before the penis is withdrawn. Apart from abstinence the use of condoms is the only way to protect oneself from HIV and STD infection. The female condom (Femidom) offers more protection in that it covers some of the vulva and it also allows women to be more in control of their own contraception and protection. In the group of women to whom I offer contraceptive advice its use has proved to be unsatisfactory. The level of skill required for its use has to be high and many drug-using women find that it is not compatible with their lifestyle. Diaphragms and cervical caps are generally not advised for such women either as, although they prevent semen reaching the cervix, they give no protection to the vagina for the prevention of STDs. Their role in HIV prevention has not been determined but the presence of an STD significantly increases the risk of transmission of HIV.

Spermicides, often used in conjunction with barrier methods, have been shown to kill HIV but if they cause allergy and inflammation of the female genital tract may, in fact, allow entry for viral infection.

Oral contraceptives

I feel that oral contraceptives may potentiate the transmission of HIV infection. Indeed chlamydia infection is increased in pill users. The pill causes columna epithelial cells to grow onto the surface of the cervix (cervical ectropion). This vulnerable tissue provides a portal of infection and again can be exacerbated by co-existing infection.

Having to take a pill every day does not fit readily into the lives of some drug-using women. The mini pill is even more problematic with the dose having to be taken at approximately the same time each day. Oestrogen-containing contraceptives have to be prescribed with caution in women drug users as oestrogens are contra-indicted if there is a history of previous cardiovascular disease. Due to injecting behaviour some will have experienced previous deep vein thromboses (DVTs) and pulmonary embolisms and so will have an adverse medical history.

Intra-uterine contraceptive device (IUD)

IUDs increase the risk of HIV transmission threefold, caused by menorrhagia and pelvic inflammatory disease associated with the use of IUD. I advise against the use of this form of contraception in female drug users.

Injectable contraceptives

Medroxydrogesterone acetate (Depo Provera) is one of the most effective contraceptives as shown in the table below. It only has to be administered every three months and fits into the lifestyles of most drug users easily. Drug agencies can even offer this service to coincide with their drug treatment counselling. Even so compliance is better than those women on oral contraceptives who often run into difficulties due to missed pills.

Table 7.1: Failure rates of contraceptives

Method	Failure rate per 100 woman years
Rhythm	16
Condom	4
IUD	3
Diaphragm	2
Mini-pill	1.2
Combined contraceptive pill	0.3
Depo-Provera injection	0.1
Female sterilization	0.1
Male sterilization	0.02

The disadvantages are that irregular periods are encountered when first commenced on the injection. Amenorrhoea may be caused by the progesterone, but is not usually considered a side effect in women who have been menstruating infrequently anyway. Once the injection has been administered any unwanted symptoms and contraceptive effect will persist for weeks until the drug has been cleared.

In a recent survey of over 200 female drug users in Liverpool, only two used more than one method of contraception. Due to the occasional failure of condoms or forgetfulness, it is advised that these women use two methods of contraception; the first to reduce the risks of HIV and a hormonal contraceptive as a safety net to prevent conception.

Social and psychological factors obviously play a major role in what contraceptive method is chosen or whether a method is used at all. Child rearing is a basic human instinct and the decision to become pregnant should be respected by the health care professional who may eventually have contact with a pregnant female user. Five per cent of female drug users are actively planning to become pregnant. Attempting to become pregnant carries with it considerable risks for a drug-using woman. A woman can only select a man to father her children from those that are available in her community. If that community has a high proportion of men who inject drugs and engage in high-risk sharing behaviour then this will be a risk to the women also. A woman will not have the opportunity to choose wisely a man who is likely to be infection-free. Before women consider pregnancy they should be made aware of the modes of transmission of HIV and given the appropriate information so that they can make informed decisions concerning the risks that are involved. Preventing the heterosexual spread of HIV in this group of women will ultimately prevent the vertical transmission of HIV from mother to child which is now globally one of the major routes of transmission.

Pre-conception care

It would be best if a drug-using woman presented before she started planning pregnancy. This is in order that her health can be stabilized to carry her pregnancy through its term without any ill effects.

Some women may be underweight and nutritionally deficient due to chaotic lifestyles, appetite suppression by illicit drugs and poverty. Dietary advice contrary to the 'normal healthy' diet of low calories and cholesterol has to be given in order to increase weight through meals containing high calories. Vitamin supplements such as multivitamins, Thianine and folic acid may need to be prescribed.

Instructing women to recognize the early signs of pregnancy and providing pregnancy testing will encourage early ante-natal booking and access to midwifery and obstetric care. It will also be an opportunity to discuss the level of women's drug use and to ascertain whether she needs to be on an oral methadone substitution programme. Many drug agencies will have priority admissions into out-patient treatment programmes. Commencing a methadone programme will help prevent women injecting and attempt to stabilize their drug use.

Table 7:2: Pre-conception investigations in female drug users

Blood tests
1. Full blood count

2. Infection screening:
a)   Rubella
b)   HBsAg and Anti HBc
c)   Serological tests for syphilis

3.Genito-urinary screening:
a)   Chlamydia
b)   High vaginal culture
c)   Cervical cytology

Blood tests will help detect nutritional anaemia and susceptibility to, and carriage of, infection. Some women in socially deprived areas may have missed the national rubella vaccination campaign for schoolgirls. Women should consider completing an accelerated Hepatitis B vaccination scheme prior to conception. Discovery of Hepatitis B carriage will be beneficial as the neonate will be offered immunoglobulin prophylaxis for protection from infection in the perinatal period. HIV testing should not be offered routinely to drug-using women as this is often perceived as discriminatory and stigmatizing. The majority of young female drug users who become pregnant have never injected and have had a monogamous relationship since coitarche, and so are not at a significantly higher risk than the general population. In areas with well developed HIV prevention services such as Liverpool, the HIV seroprevalence is extremely low and the costs incurred in routine HIV testing are not justified.

It would be advantageous for a woman to have a full sexual health screening in a GUM clinic. In a survey of female attendees at the Liverpool Drug Dependency Clinic a fifth had previously had an abnormal smear test with nearly a third never having had a smear. This suggests that there is a significant risk in this population and that they require vigilant surveillance. Any treatment required or further investigation should be completed before pregnancy.

Some women who become pregnant may wish not to continue with it. Eight per cent of drug-using women who become pregnant eventually have a termination of pregnancy. They may feel their drug use is not sufficiently well controlled or their social circumstances have deteriorated to such an extent it is inappropriate to care for a child in such an environment.

Therefore, women should have access to abortion services. Even in some parts of Liverpool discrimination exists as drug-using women do not have access to NHS abortion services. If the woman has the child it results in increased psychological costs of social service involvement, often requested by the women themselves, to provide statutory child care.

About the author
Dr Clive L. Morrison is a vocational trained General Practitioner and has worked for four years in substance misuse and HIV prevention. In his role as Senior Clinical Medical Officer for Special Groups he provides family health care for drug users, prostitutes and HIV positive people. He has a unique expertise in the management of the complications of injecting drug misuse.

He has a special interest in the care and prescribing of methadone to pregnant drug users within the Liverpool Drug Dependency Clinic. Another role is to liaise between the local GUM and Drug Dependency services. He has collaborated in many research projects with other allied health professionals including the Regional Infectious Diseases Unit with a particular emphasis on the health care needs of drug users.

CHAPTER EIGHT

Sexually Transmitted Diseases, Pregnancy and the Drug User

PETER CAREY

The sexually transmitted diseases (STDs) are a group of contagious conditions whose principal mode of transmission is by intimate sexual activity involving the moist mucous membranes of the penis, vulva, vagina, cervix, anus, rectum, mouth and throat and their adjacent areas of skin. Departments of Genitourinary Medicine (GUM) throughout the UK continue to be pivotal in their diagnosis and treatment.

Some of the principles involved in the management of these infections include:

1. accurate diagnosis;
2. effective treatment;
3. investigations to establish cure before resumption of sexual activity;
4. partner notification (contact tracing) to prevent further spread of infection in the community or reinfection of the index case;
5. counselling around safer sexual practices;
6. the exhibition of a confidential, friendly, well advertised and easily accessible environment for patient care.

Whilst a variety of microorganisms have the potential for sexual spread I intend to concentrate on those outlined below. Standard treatments may have to be changed in pregnancy because of the potential for fetal damage and there may be poor compliance in drug users if treatment is prolonged.

Bacterial infections:
*   Syphilis
*   Gonorrhoea
*   Chlamydial infection
*   Organisms associated with bacterial vaginosis
*   Group B streptococci

Viral infections:
* Genital herpes
* Genital warts

Protozoal infection:
* Trichomoniasis

Fungal infection:
* Vaginal candidosis

Ectoparasites:
* Scabies
* Pubic lice

Infections associated with hepatitis B virus (HBV), hepatitis C virus (HCV) and human immunodeficiency virus (HIV) are dealt with in separate chapters.

Space does not allow for lengthy description of each infection and this chapter is not intended as a 'do-it-yourself' guide.

Altered cell mediated immunity in pregnancy may modify the course of certain STDs. Some STDs may be associated with spontaneous abortion, stillbirth, congenital abnormalities or perinatal infection, whilst ectopic pregnancy or infertility may be a consequence of previous salpingitis associated with gonococcal or chlamydial infections.

The pregnant drug user may be at special risk of STDs if she has to earn money in the sex industry or exchange sexual favours for drugs. The effect of certain drugs may influence her sexual behaviour or her partner's, if he uses drugs. If she continues to share injecting equipment she puts herself at potential risk of HBV, HCV or HIV infection. These and other health problems associated with sharing injecting equipment are dealt with elsewhere in this book.

Syphilis

Syphilis is caused by infection with Treponema pallidum. Following an incubation period of about three weeks (range 9–90 days) a painless indurated ulcer, the chancre (Fig. 8.1), develops at the site of inoculation of the treponemes, usually on the vulva but sometimes on the cervix. Genital lesions are associated with the painless enlargement or superficial inguinal glands. Extra-genital chancres have been described on the lips (Fig. 8.2), tongue, nipple and finger. Transmission is usually sexual or from mother to baby. Accidental infection is very rare.

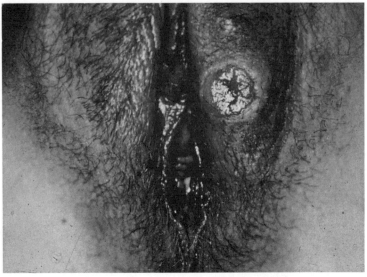

Fig. 8.1: Chancre – right labium majus

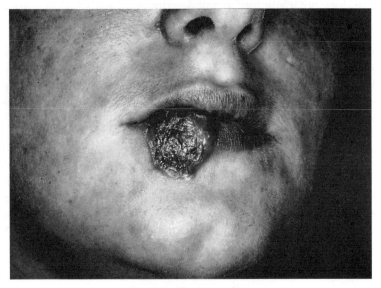

Fig. 8.2: Chancre – lip

This is the stage of primary syphilis. Without treatment the chancre slowly heals to be followed by secondary syphilis about two months later (Fig. 8.3), due to the widespread dissemination of treponemes throughout the body. Characteristically a widespread symmetrical, non-irritable maculopapular rash develops involving all body surfaces. Mucosal lesions (snail track ulcers) may be seen in the mouth whilst hypertrophic papules (condylomata lata) may develop at sites of the body liable to friction and maceration, e.g. genital area (Fig. 8.4).

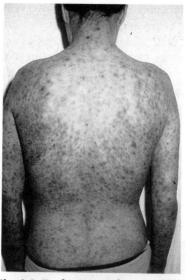

Fig. 8.3: Rash – secondary syphilis

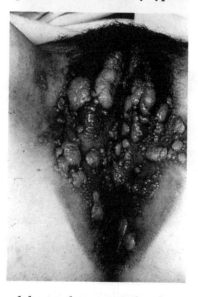

Fig. 8.4: Condylomata lata – genital and perianal areas

Other symptoms such as headache, fever and malaise are included in a range of protean manifestations. Without treatment this stage resolves, entering the stage of early latency which ends arbitrarily, two years after infection. Thereafter late latency exists which may continue unchanged for life or be terminated by the development of some form of tertiary syphilis: gummatous disease (benign tertiary syphilis), cardiovascular syphilis or neurosyphilis.

People are sexually infectious during the first two years or so after infection. Mothers who have untreated primary or secondary syphilis during pregnancy will infect their babies transplacentally or perinatally, depending on the timing of infection. Untreated they remain able to infect their babies for many years thereafter with the risk reducing over time. Treatment of mother during pregnancy allows for treatment of her fetus in utero as penicillin crosses the placenta.

Consequences for pregnancy and baby

Overwhelming intrauterine infection leads to spontaneous abortion, stillbirth or the premature birth, or birth at term, of a very sick baby with clinical signs of early congenital syphilis (see Fig. 8.5).

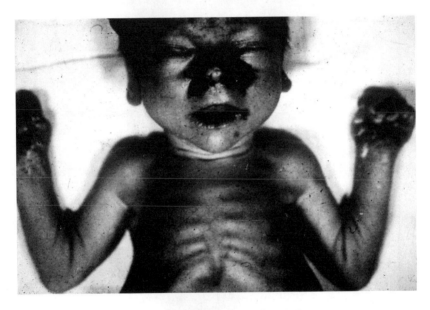

Fig. 8.5: Early congenital syphilis

Infection near term or peripartum may be associated with the development of signs of early congenital syphilis during the first few weeks of life (Fig. 8.6) or a baby who has latent infection but who may develop late congenital syphilis and associated stigmata, later in life.

Diagnosis

Treponemes may be found in serum collected from chancres. Serum from moist or eroded lesions in secondary syphilis and similar lesions from babies with early congenital syphilis may also yield treponemes.

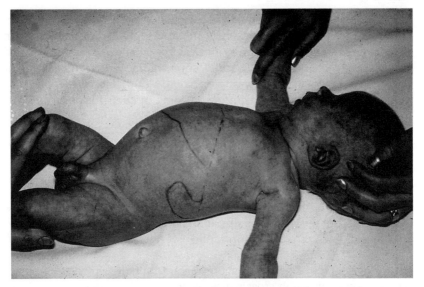

Fig. 8.6: Early congenital syphilis – hepatosplenomegaly

Syphilis serology	RPR	:	Rapid Plasma Reagin Test
or	VDRL	:	Venereal Disease Research Laboratory Test
	TPHA	:	Treponema Pallidum Haema-glutination Assay
	FTA ABS	:	Fluorescent Treponemal Anti-body Absorption Test.

These tests are positive in people with treponemal infections and do not differentiate syphilis from non-venereal treponemal infections such as yaws. The RPR or VDRL are non-treponemal tests. They may give false positive results in some people when TPHA and FTA ABS tests will be negative.

Increasing seropositivity is seen for RPR, TPHA and FTA ABS through the primary and secondary stages reaching a maximum in the late secondary stage. Thereafter titres decline slowly over time, even without treatment.

Passively transferred maternal antibody from a treated mother to her baby leads to seropositivity which declines to negative during the first six months of life. Stable or increasing titres in baby equate with infection, treatment of the baby and further investigation of mother.

Treatment

Mothers are treated with a course of intramuscular procaine penicillin appropriate to the stage of syphilis. Resolution of clinical lesions and declining syphilis serology titres equate with good response to treatment.

Jarish-Herxheimer reaction should be anticipated and explained to mother. It is common on day 1 of treatment in early syphilis (but may occur in other stages) and is due to rapid killing of treponemes; fever, malaise and headache are characteristic. Uterine contractions, premature labour or reduced fetal movements may be associated. Mothers should report these immediately. It has been my custom to admit mothers for observation at the initiation of treatment.

Babies with early congenital syphilis are admitted to hospital for treatment with either intramuscular procaine penicillin or intravenous benzyl penicillin. Follow up after treatment is for two years.

A mother who has had an anaphylactic reaction with penicillin should be treated with erythromycin. As this antibiotic crosses the placenta poorly, her baby should be treated with a course of penicillin following delivery.

For lesser degrees of penicillin allergy an appropriate cephalosporin may be substituted, although cross reactions between the two antibiotics have been reported. Partner and other children should be investigated and treated if syphilis is found.

Gonorrhoea

Gonorrhoea is usually acquired sexually. The causative organisms, Neiserria gonorrhoea (gonococci) are delicate and have limited ability to remain viable outside the body. However, they can survive in purulent discharge on towels for some hours and so accidental mucosal infection is possible.

Gonococci infect mucosal surfaces because of their affinity for columnar epithelium, with resulting submucosal inflammation and marked neutrophil response. Urethra (Fig. 8.7), para-urethral ducts, Bartholin's ducts (Fig. 8.8), endocervical canal (Fig. 8.9), rectum (Fig. 8.10), pharynx or eyes may be affected sites. Infection may be asymptomatic in many women though some may complain of dysuria or altered vaginal discharge, usually within ten days of infection. Rectal or pharyngeal infections may be silent whilst gonococcal conjunctivitis is painful and purulent.

Clinical examination may be unremarkable or show purulent exudate from urethra, para-urethral ducts or Bartholin's ducts, or mucopurulent discharge from the endocervical canal, with erythema of cervical ectopy. The rectum may show evidence of proctitis with erythema and mucopus. Evidence of pharyngitis or tonsillitis is usually lacking. Rectal infection may be associated with receptive anal sex though more often due to contamination by vaginal discharge containing gonococci. Pharyngeal infection occurs from oral penile contact. If eyes are infected, by contamination from infected fingers, for instance, purulent conjunctivitis with erythema and oedema will be in evidence.

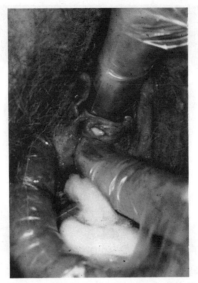

Fig. 8.7: Gonococcal infection – urethra

Presumptive diagnosis is made on microscopy by finding gonococci as gram negative intracellular diplococci on gram stained smears taken from one or more of the above sites. Pharyngeal smears are not examined because other Neiserrian organisms here may confuse the picture. Microscopy is about 60 per cent sensitive in diagnosing gonorrhoea in women and so swabs from these sites, including pharynx, are inoculated on to selective media to be cultured in a warm, carbon dioxide enriched environment. Specific identification using monoclonal antibodies, and antibiotic sensitivities, follow successful culture.

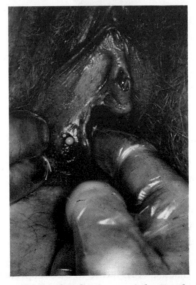

Fig. 8.8: Gonococcal infection – right Bartholin's duct

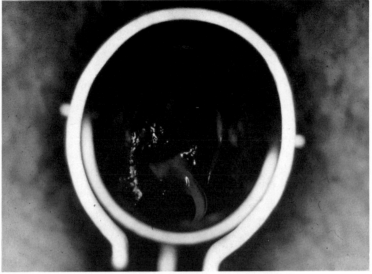

Fig. 8.9: Gonococcal infection – cervix

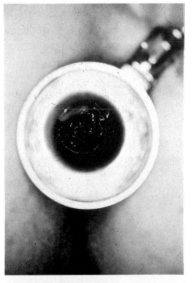

Fig. 8.10: Gonococcal infection – rectum

Pregnancy complications

Gonococcal infection may be associated with:

1. premature rupture of membranes;
2. chorioamnionitis;
3. premature delivery.

Pelvic inflammatory disease (PID), due to direct spread of gonococci from endocervical canal to infect uterine cavity and fallopian tubes, is rare in pregnancy. It may occur early but presumably the hostile environment in endocervical mucus and the obliteration of the uterine cavity at the 16th week of pregnancy by the gestational sac, have protective effects. Untreated gonorrhoea may be associated with post-partum endometritis.

Disseminated gonococcal infection (DGI) associated with pustular skin lesions, arthralgia and then septic arthritis is thought to be more common in pregnancy.

Infection of baby

Intrapartum infections give rise to gonococcal ophthalmia neonatorum (Fig. 8.11) in about 50 per cent of babies.

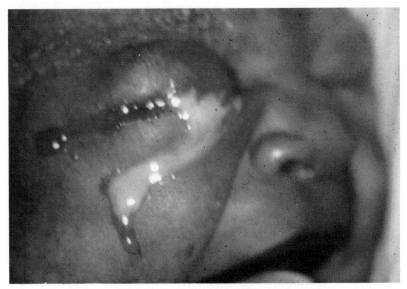

Fig. 8.11: Gonococcal ophthalmia neonatorum

Presentation is usually within 48 hours of birth as a purulent conjunctivitis with oedema of eyelids. One or both eyes may be involved. Diagnosis is made by finding gonococci in gram stained smears and from culture of ocular pus. Pharyngeal swab should also be taken for culture. Delay in diagnosis may lead to serious corneal involvement and possibly blindness. DGI is rare.

Management of the mother

Single dose treatments are satisfactory for uncomplicated gonococcal infection. Some strains of gonococci are penicillin resistant and this should be remembered when selecting an appropriate antibiotic. Regimes based on penicillins and probenecid, cephalosporins or spectinomycin are safe to use in pregnancy, when treatments based on ciprofloxacin are contraindicated. Some women may be infected also with chlamydia to which these antibiotics have no efficacy. Erythromycin is a suitable addition to treatment in this circumstance.

Following treatment of mother two negative tests of cure are required and her partner must be investigated and treated.

Complicated gonococcal infection during pregnancy should be managed in hospital with more prolonged antibiotic therapy appropriate to the complication. PID, DGI and gonococcal conjunctivitis all have serious implications for health.

Management of the baby

Treatment regimes vary but tend to be based on systemic cephalosporins. When one eye is infected the other should be protected with an eyepatch. The affected eye(s) should be irrigated with buffered saline every hour until the purulent discharge settles. Tests of cure follow treatment. DGI will require prolonged antibiotic treatment.

Chlamydial infection

Chlamydia trachomatis (chlamydia) is an intracellular bacterium with a predilection for infecting columnar epithelium. Submucosal inflammation and neutrophil response characterize infection. Both chlamydia and gonococci infect similar sites of the body and infections may coexist. Chlamydial infection usually results from sexual or perinatal transmission.

For many women infection is asymptomatic though some may complain of dysuria or vaginal discharge. Urethral infection may be associated with sterile pyuria whilst cervical infection may produce mucopurulent cervicitis. Conversely both sites may be infected without clinical signs. In practice most women are diagnosed by the detection of chlamydial antigen from endocervical swabs using ELISA and fluorescent antibody tests.

Pregnancy complications

Chlamydial infection may be associated with:

1.   preterm premature rupture of membranes;
2.   preterm delivery;
3.   preterm labour;
4.   low birthweight.

PID is uncommon in pregnancy. Chlamydial infection may be associated with reactive arthropathy or tenosynovitis, or Reiter's disease: the combination or urethritis or cervicitis, conjunctivitis or iritis, arthritis and mucocutaneous lesions. These complications are far less common in women than in men.

Untreated chlamydial infection in pregnancy may be associated with postpartum endometritis.

Infection of baby

Intrapartum infection is associated with chlamydial ophthalmia neonatorum in about 40 per cent of babies, usually developing five days or more after delivery. Clinical signs in the eye(s) may be similar to gonococcal ophthalmia neonatorum but in some, infection may be minimal.

The oropharynx may be colonized, with possible infection of the middle ear or descending infection to produce pneumonitis. The latter may develop within six weeks of birth, presenting as a staccato cough with tachypnoea and interstitial shadowing on chest X-ray.

Management

Erythromycin is the antibiotic of choice for treating chlamydial infection in pregnancy. One week's treatment is prescribed for uncomplicated infection. The estolate preparation should be avoided because of its association with hepatotoxicity in pregnancy. Tests of cure follow four weeks after completing treatment. Her partner should be investigated and treated.

Erythromycin syrup for two weeks is effective treatment for both chlamydial ophthalmia neonatorum and chlamydial pneumonitis. Tests of cure as above.

Bacterial vaginosis

Bacterial vaginosis (BV) is usually found in sexually active women though whether it should be regarded as a sexually transmitted disease remains controversial. The hydrogen peroxide producing lactobacilli in the vagina are replaced by a variety of microorganisms such as Gardnerella vaginalis, Bacteroides and Mobilunci species or Mycoplasma hominis. The mechanism for this is incompletely understood.

The characteristic complaint of offensive vaginal discharge, often having a 'fishy' odour and worse after sexual intercourse, is found in about 50 per cent of affected women. Clinical examination reveals a thin, white homogenous discharge presenting on the vulva, vaginal walls and cervix.

As there is no associated inflammatory response, vulvitis, vaginitis and cervicitis are absent, though BV organisms may be associated with PID.

Diagnosis of BV is based on finding three out of the four following symptoms:

1.   characteristic vaginal discharge;
2.   vaginal pH > 4.5;
3.   fishy amine odour following application of ten per cent potassium hydroxide to vaginal discharge on a microscope slide;
4.   clue cells: desquamated vaginal epithelial cells whose borders are obscured by large numbers of BV organisms as viewed microscopically.

Pregnancy complications
BV has been linked with:

1.   chorioamnionitis;
2.   preterm rupture of membranes;
3.   preterm delivery;
4.   postpartum endometritis.

Management
Metronidazole is the treatment of choice for BV in non-pregnant women and has been used for the treatment of BV in the second and third trimesters of pregnancy. The introduction of clindamycin 2% vaginal cream for BV treatment provides a satisfactory alternative in pregnancy. Further studies are required to define the effect of either treatment in reducing pregnancy complications. Relapse after treatment may occur and research tends to suggest that epidemiological treatment of sexual partners will not prevent this (McGregor et al, 1994).

Group B streptococcus (GBS)
Vaginal colonization by GBS may occur in up to 25 per cent of pregnant women, with up to 75 per cent of neonates acquiring GBS from their mothers intrapartum. Of these, 0.5–1 per cent develop disseminated GBS disease with a mortality of 50 per cent (Adimora et al, 1994).

GBS may be grown from swabs taken from urethra, vagina and rectum and cultured from urine. Neonatal swabs are taken from ears, nose, pharynx rectum and umbilicus.

Pregnancy complications

1.   Premature rupture of membranes.
2.   Prolonged rupture of membranes.
3.   Intrapartum fever.
4.   Post-partum endometritis.

Management

Various strategies have been explored to prevent GBS infection in neonates. Immunisation of mothers against GBS infection is being researched whilst intrapartum treatment of GBS infected mothers with intravenous antibiotics has been shown to be effective in reducing GBS transmission to neonates (Katz et al, 1994). Prophylactic antibiotic treatment of GBS exposed neonates has also been studied.

Treatment of mother and her partner during pregnancy is ineffective because of subsequent recolonization of the vagina by GBS.

Genital herpes

Herpes simplex virus (HSV) infection of the genital tract results from sexual contact with an individual shedding virus from mucosa or skin. In many cases the source may be unaware of his or her infection. Accidental infection from HSV contaminated fomites seems to be rare as virus survives for only a short time outside the body.

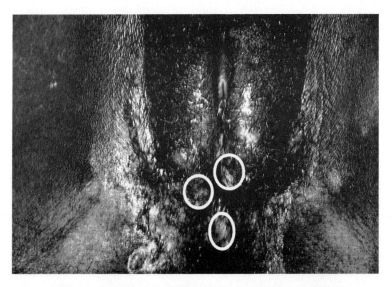

Fig. 8.12: Genital herpes (with some ulcers circled)

Historically HSV-1 has been associated with 'cold sores' on the lips (herpes labialis) and HSV-2 with genital infection, but HSV-1 has been found in genital infection and HSV-2 in oropharyngeal infection. The majority of genital infections are associated with HSV-2.

In the UK there have been increasing numbers of people presenting with genital herpes during the last decade. Research in the USA suggests that 75 per cent of people with antibodies to HSV-2, indicative of previous infection, have no antecedent history of symptomatic disease.

Primary infection establishes HSV in mucous membranes or skin, followed by local replication. Herpes simplex virus is neurotropic entering sensory nerve endings in the infected site and travelling along the nerve to the dorsal root ganglion. This mechanism establishes latency. Following recovery from primary infection recurrences may follow due to reactivation of HSV in the ganglion. Virus travels along the sensory nerve to produce further infection of mucous membrane or skin. This may lead to clinical recurrence or symptomless virus shedding.

The mechanisms for establishing latency and recurrences are not clearly understood. 'Triggering' factors are thought to play a part in reactivation of virus such as fever, trauma, anxiety, sexual intercourse, menstruation or exposure to ultraviolet light.

The chance of recurrence during the first year from infection is thought to be 60 per cent for HSV-1 and 90 per cent for HSV-2.

Sites of infection
1.   Vulva, urethra, vagina, cervix.
2.   Perineum.
3.   Perianal area, rectum.
4.   Oropharynx.
5.   Other sites: buttocks, finger, eyes.

Clinical presentation
Symptomatic primary infection with HSV-2 produces marked local and systemic symptoms which are less severe in those who have experienced previous infection with HSV-1. The incubation period is usually within seven days of infection. Following vulval irritation vesicles develop which then ulcerate. The area involved may be extensive and involve vulva and perianal area. Genital pain is characteristic with marked dysuria, either due to urethral infection or urine contact with genital ulcers. Superficial inguinal glands are likely to be enlarged and tender. Fever is common

with headache and myalgia. Aseptic meningitis complicates a proportion of cases. Rarely autonomic dysfunction is encountered presenting with urinary retention and a large atonic bladder. This should not be confused with the avoidance of micturition in women with severe genital herpes, particularly with urethral involvement, when it becomes too painful to pass urine.

Oropharyngeal infection may be associated with erythema or ulceration of the palate or pharynx with associated tender cervical lymphadenopathy.

Other non-genital sites of infection include buttock, finger or eye(s). Such lesions develop later and are probably the result of autoinoculation of HSV from genital lesions.

Healing takes place over two to three weeks with crusting of skin lesions and re-epithelialization of mucosal lesions. Secondary bacterial infection is uncommon but vaginal discharge may be prominent in the presence of herpetic cervicitis. The cervix is infected in up to 90 per cent of primary episodes: vaginal candidosis may coexist.

Recurrences are less extensive or severe compared with primary episodes with resolution of lesions within seven to ten days. Recurrence rates vary between individuals.

Diagnosis
Swabs from herpetic lesions are sent in transport medium to the laboratory. Positive results from tissue culture are available within 48 to 72 hours. Direct electron microscopy for herpes virus in smears from lesions may be available in some laboratories. This investigation will not differentiate herpes simplex viruses from other herpes viruses such as Varicella zoster virus.

At present most laboratories are unable to detect antibodies specific for HSV-1 or HSV-2 and so individuals who are infected asymptomatically with these viruses cannot be differentiated. The Herpes simplex virus complement fixation test (HSCFT) is universally available but does not differentiate between HSV-1 and HSV-2. Its value is in the diagnosis or primary infection when seroconversion and rising titre will be seen.

Management
The principles involved should address:

1. protecting women who have not previously experienced genital herpes from partners who have either histories of genital or orolabial herpes;

2.   preventing peripartum HSV infection or neonates from mothers with histories of genital herpes, mothers with exposure to HSV during pregnancy or mothers with primary genital herpes particularly during the last trimester or at term;

3.   preventing post-partum HSV infection of babies from parents or attendants with labial or orolabial herpes.

Detailed advice is beyond the scope of this chapter but may be outlined as follows.

Protecting mother

Abstinence from sexual intercourse (rarely possible) or consistent use for HSV discordant couples to protect mother from acquiring infection during pregnancy.

Counselling about risks of HSV transmission from oral-genital contact for male partners with a history of labial or orolabial herpes.

Management during pregnancy

Although not licensed for use in pregnancy acyclovir has been prescribed for pregnant women with distressing symptomatic genital herpes. So far no teratogenic or toxic fetal effects have been associated with such use.

Management of delivery

Caesarean section, within four hours of rupture of membranes, is advised for women with primary genital herpes at term. Their genital herpes should be treated with acyclovir. If this cannot be achieved and the decision is to deliver vaginally intrapartum treatment with intravenous acyclovir, followed by postpartum treatment for both mother and baby, should be given.

Similarly Caesarean section is recommended at 38 weeks gestation for women who have experienced primary genital herpes during the third trimester.

Caesarean section should also be considered for women with recurrence of genital herpes at term or who experience frequent recurrences during pregnancy.

Women at risk from HSV infection during pregnancy should be examined for genital herpes at ANC visits and swabs taken for confirmatory culture from suspicious lesions. If primary genital herpes develops during the third trimester or at term, management procedures outlined above should be followed. Women with primary episodes before the third trimester may deliver vaginally if there is no recurrence at term.

Women with histories of genital herpes should deliver vaginally unless herpetic lesions are present at term.

Despite these precautions neonates will still be infected by mothers with no prior history of genital herpes who shed virus asymptomatically at term. This is likely to produce strong feelings of guilt in mothers who will require expert counselling.

Management of baby

Babies born vaginally to mothers with genital herpes should have swabs taken for HSV from eyes, oropharynx and areas of skin trauma. Note that trauma to baby from instruments or scalp electrodes during delivery may increase the risk of neonatal HSV infection.

Treatment with intravenous acyclovir should be given to:

- babies with positive HSV cultures;
- babies with clinical signs of HSV infection.

Prophylactic acyclovir should be given to babies born vaginally to mothers with primary genital herpes at term and considered for babies born vaginally to mothers with recurrences at term.

Prevention of postnatal infection

Parents, other family members or staff with orolabial infections should be counselled about the possible risk of HSV transmission to baby. Mothers with HSV lesions on their breasts should not breastfeed their babies.

Close liaison between Obstetric team and GUM Physician is essential for the proper coordination of care.

Genital warts

The sexual transmission of Human papilloma virus (HPV) may produce a disease spectrum ranging from sub-clinical genital tract infection to overt clinical disease characterized by genital warts. It is not known how frequently genital HPV infection is acquired non-sexually.

HPV DNA typing has demonstrated more than 70 genotypes. HPV 6 and 11 are most commonly associated with anogenital warts whilst HPV 16, 18 and 31 are associated with cervical intraepithelial neoplasia and invasive squamous cell carcinoma of the cervix.

Disease spectrum

1. Sub-clinical infection in the genital tract.
2. Clinically obvious warts affecting vulva, vagina, cervix, perineum or anus.
3. Koilocytes on cervical cytology.
4. Vulval, vaginal or cervical intraepithelium neoplasia (VIN, VAIN, CIN).
5. Bowenoid papulosis.
6. Oral warts.

The incubation period for the development of genital warts is up to six months, possibly more, following sexual acquisition of HPV. It is not known whether there is any difference in sexual infectivity between individuals who have warts in the genital tract compared with those sub-clinically infected with HPV.

At present it is not possible to eradicate HPV from the genital tract and so the aim of treatment is to remove visible warts.

HPV and pregnancy

HPV infection does not appear to have any adverse effect on pregnancy outcome but genital warts may increase in size and number. In some instances the degree of HPV associated CIN has worsened.

HPV and baby

There is an association between the development of juvenile laryngeal papillomata and the presence of HPV in the maternal genital tract at delivery. Infection is peripartum and uncommon. Peripartum HPV infection of the anogenital area of the baby may also be a rare occurrence. It should be remembered that the development of anogenital warts in a baby may be associated with sexual abuse.

Management

Genital warts are usually treated with podophyllin or podophyllotoxin preparations which are contraindicated in pregnancy. Treatment with the CO_2 cryoprobe or liquid nitrogen may be effective as may the careful topical application of 90% trichloroacetic acid. This preparation should be used with great care as painful skin ulceration may be the result of overenthusiastic use. Irrespective of treatment choice a small number of warts should be treated initially to assess response. It has been my practice to restrict the use of trichloroacetic acid to external warts only.

Biopsy is recommended if the diagnosis of genital warts is in doubt and should be considered before the treatment of anogenital warts in babies if sexual abuse is a possibility.

The treatment of genital warts in babies requires the close cooperation of mother and clinic staff. CO_2 cryotherapy is time-consuming and therefore difficult in practice. Careful electrodesiccation of warts, following local anaesthesia, may be useful.

Prevention
Caesarean section is not recommended to prevent HPV infection in baby. However, it may be necessary if genital warts become so extensive as to obstruct labour or prevent episiotomy (Fig. 8.13). This complication is fortunately rare. Biopsy may be required to exclude malignancy.

Regular condom use may be successful in preventing HPV acquisition for some men but HPV may infect the genital area which remains unprotected during sexual intercourse.

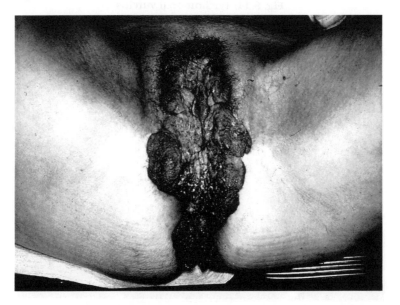

Fig. 8.13: Extensive genital warts in pregnancy

Trichomoniasis

Infection with the protozoon Trichomonas vaginalis (TV) may be associated with vulvitis (Fig. 8.14), vaginitis and cervicitis (Fig. 8.15).

Vulval pruritus, vaginal discharge and dysuria are the main complains. A proportion of women have no associated symptoms.

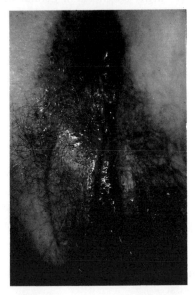

Fig. 8.14: Trichomonal vulvitis

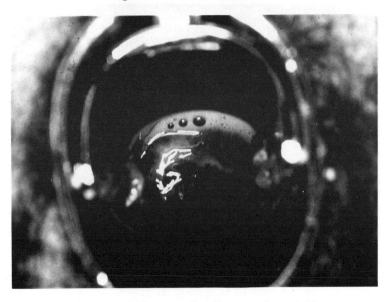

Fig. 8.15: Trichomonal vaginitis and cervicitis

TV infection is usually acquired sexually though non-sexually acquired infection has been reported. Diagnosis is made by finding the characteristically motile trichomonads on microscopy of a wet preparation of vaginal discharge in the presence of neutrophils. TV may be cultured from vaginal swabs inoculated into Feinberg Whittington medium.

Management

Metronidazole is the treatment of choice for TV infections but debate continues about its safety in pregnancy. Clotrimazole vaginal cream has some anti-trichomonal activity and may be used in the first trimester with metronidazole reserved for treatment of trichomoniasis in the second and third trimesters.

In some people metronidazole has a disulfiram-like action when alcoholic beverages are drunk and may produce headaches, flushing, nausea or vomiting. Mothers should be warned not to drink alcohol when taking metronidazole.

Male partners, who may be asymptomatic, should be investigated and treated.

Pregnancy complications

Research data suggest that vaginal trichomoniasis may be associated with preterm delivery.

Intrapartum transmission to a female baby with vaginal colonization is said to be uncommon.

Vaginal candidosis

Vulvo-vaginal candidosis is seen commonly in women during their reproductive years, about 20 per cent carrying Candida species in the genital tract. The majority of yeasts isolated from the vagina are Candida albicans. Factors predisposing to symptomatic disease include pregnancy, diabetes mellitus, antibiotic therapy and local factors such as close fitting nylon underwear. The bowel may be a source for recurring candidal infection in some women. Sexual transmission may also be a source of infection, though difficult to prove.

Vulval pruritis, with or without vaginal discharge, is the usual presentation. Vulvitis is obvious on clinical examination with vaginal erythema and usually a white caseous discharge. In pregnancy symptoms are said to be more severe and episodes more frequent.

Peter Carey

Diagnosis
Microscopic examination of a wet preparation of vaginal discharge may reveal the characteristic morphology of the yeast whilst culture is the most sensitive diagnostic test. Testing urine for glucose should be routine.

Management
Candidosis in pregnancy is seldom associated with complications though cases of chorioamnionitis have been described. Frequent relapses warrant investigation for predisposing causes remembering that recurrent genital candidosis may be a feature of HIV-1 infection in some women.

Topical treatments based on clotrimazole, miconazole or econazole creams are commonly used and effective. Systemic treatments with fluconazole and itraconazole are contraindicated. The partner should be treated if balanitis is present and consideration given to epidemiological treatment should recurrences of vulvovaginitis present.

Perinatal infection of baby may be associated with oral candidosis in the genital area. Nystatin suspension is suitable for oral infection with topical treatment to the involved skin. Nystatin cream or clotrimazole cream may be used.

Scabies
Infection with Sarcoptes scabiei has no effect on pregnancy, fetus or baby and is acquired either sexually or from close body contact with an infected individual. Pruritus, worse at night, develops about one month after infection but much earlier in those who have been infected previously. Treatment with topical benzyl benzoate is the treatment of choice, the more commonly prescribed 1% lindane being contraindicated in pregnancy. Sexual partner and close family members should also be treated.

Pubic lice (Pediculosis pubis)
Infestation with Phthirus pubis (the 'crab louse') has no consequences for pregnancy, fetus or baby. Pubic, perianal, axillary and other coarse body hair may be involved. Rarely eyebrows or eyelashes may be sites affected.

Standard treatment with 1% lindane is contraindicated in pregnancy. If infestation is sparse individual lice and eggs (nits) may be picked off. Heavier infestation may be treated with the topical application of 0.5% malathion as an aqueous lotion. This preparation should not be used near the eyes where applications of occlusive ophthalmic ointment should be used for infestation of eyelashes or eyebrows.

Traditional recommendations to launder recently used underwear and bedlinen apply in the management of both scabies and pubic lice.

Safer sex

If you don't have a sexual infection and your partner doesn't, sexual intercourse is 'safe', i.e. there is no infection within the relationship to transmit sexually. Many people don't possess these facts about themselves or their partners and for them safer sex means the use of condoms to protect against infection. Their consistent use before any genital contact is made should be emphasized. Following ejaculation the condom should be held firmly around the erect penis during withdrawal, to prevent leakage of semen.

Condoms are also recommended for oral-penile sex with flavoured varieties available. Dental dams, thin squares of latex rubber (also flavoured) have been suggested for application to the vulva, prior to and during, oral-vulval sex, so protecting two potential sites of infection.

Safer sex may not sound very romantic but neither is the acquisition of a sexually transmitted disease!

Further information about safer sex may be obtained from your local GUM Clinic (see below).

Conclusion

Regular screening of women at risk of STDs will help to reduce the prevalence of these conditions in pregnancy. The diagnosis of one STD necessitates investigations for others. GUM Clinics are best equipped for this task.

Routine testing for syphilis should continue in antenatal clinics and be repeated later in pregnancy, if new STDs are discovered.

Repeat screening for STDs in pregnancy should be considered for women who may be having unprotected sex with different partners. The consistent practice of safer sex will complement screening for STDs.

There is a comprehensive network of GUM clinics throughout the UK with enthusiastic medical staff, nursing staff and health advisers available to give advice in person, by telephone or to act as a source of referral for patients with a wide range of sexual health problems. A list of GUM clinics in the UK can be obtained by telephoning 0800 665544.

About the author

Dr Peter Carey qualified at Liverpool University in 1970. He is a Fellow of the Royal College of Physicians and has been a consultant in Genitourinary Medicine in Liverpool for 16 years. He has developed a specialist interest in HIV medicine during the last 11 years. He has outpatient and inpatient responsibilities in the Royal Liverpool and Broadgreen University Hospital NHS Trust together with a contribution to community care. He is an honorary lecturer at Liverpool University.

CHAPTER NINE

Outreach Work with Female Sex Workers in Liverpool

LYN MATTHEWS

The emergence of AIDS as the major health concern during the latter part of this century has forced us to reconsider a number of assumptions about the society we live in. Individual lifestyles, sexual practices and drug using behaviour have all been exposed in the light of a tragedy which continues to unfold. Moral concerns compete with a public health agenda which aims to prevent the spread of a virus which threatens us all, and thereby staggers efforts to protect our communities. Despite this, common sense and compassion can often prevail, albeit for a limited period, in the most desperate of circumstances. The following describes part of my work with prostitutes in Liverpool during the years of 1987 to 1992

Background

In October 1986 the Mersey Regional Drugs Training and Information Centre initiated an injecting equipment exchange scheme in Liverpool as an attempt to prevent the spread of HIV through the sharing of used needles and syringes by local drug users. At this time Merseyside, and in particular Liverpool, was being singled out in the media as an area of particularly high levels of heroin use and, because of this, the city was divided on how to tackle the problem. While local politicians played on community fears and called for ever more draconian measures to punish individual drug users, health workers took a more pragmatic stance by attempting to address the issue from a much broader public health perspective. Despite the very real threat posed by AIDS, giving needles to drug users was considered highly controversial and, in the words of one community activist, on a par with 'giving guns to murderers'. In hindsight, the 'radical' or 'controversial' nature of this approach, which has since been adopted worldwide, now seems exactly what it was to us at the time – common sense.

To avoid a media backlash and public over-reaction, the cooperation of the police and local newspaper were secured on the basis that this 'experiment', although in the best interests of society, may not even get off the ground. Injecting drug users are a marginalized and, consequently, highly suspicious group and to attract them into the scheme a user-friendly, non-judgmental approach was needed. To advertise the service, news of its location was spread by word of mouth in the first instance. Although hampered by an almost covert operational policy and with minimal staffing, word of the initiative travelled quickly among drug users and the scheme began attracting clients from the city and outlying areas. In the first six weeks of operation over 300 people came in to exchange used needles and syringes.

As well as supplying clean injecting equipment, staff at the centre also provided free condoms and advice on safer sex. Among the women attending the scheme were a number of female sex workers who also injected drugs. Initial discussions with these women revealed that sex workers operating in a particular area, near to the city centre, were experiencing difficulties in obtaining sufficient supplies of condoms for their needs. Consequently, it was decided to supply these women with enough condoms to last them a week or more, free of charge. However, these women told their non-injecting colleagues of the scheme and soon they too requested supplies of free condoms. The uptake of this service highlighted that although specific knowledge of HIV infection was scant, these women were sufficiently concerned by what they had gleaned from media reporting to take the issue seriously.

Initial work with the women led to the realization that a number of strategies needed to be adopted in order to develop a coherent approach to the prevention of HIV infection among this group. These included problem definition, information gathering, and the identification of specific practical policies.

The first step was to clarify the problem and define the target population. From informal discussions with the women using the syringe exchange scheme, it became clear that many of their clients were insisting on oral, vaginal, and anal sex without barrier protection. If a women refused to do 'business' without a condom, many of the men (or 'mushes' as they were called by the women) would drive on until they found a women who would. Given the fact that people engage in prostitution to make money, many women reported giving in to such requests. Also, the women's knowledge of HIV/AIDS and other infections, such as Hepatitis B, was poor and in the main based on information gleaned from the mass media, much of which was confused, contradictory, or inaccurate.

It soon became apparent that immediate intervention was needed and more detailed information was required in order to formulate and develop constructive prevention programmes. To this end, it was decided that condoms should be made more readily available and information concerning sexual health should be disseminated. It was also felt that contact should be made with more women working within the sex industry, although it was unclear how this goal could be achieved.

An early attempt to invite a group of women to a meeting to discuss AIDS prevention was a complete failure. No one attended. Traditionally, women working within the sex industry have received short shrift from straight society and are suspicious of statutory services of all kinds. One of the women explained why the meeting failed, 'We thought it would be full of social worker types' and, of course, she was quite right. Waiting to greet them at this meeting, alongside a neatly laid out cold buffet, were various dignitaries from the Regional Health Authority including the head of the Health Promotion Unit and his secretary, the Drugs and HIV Coordinator, the consultant psychiatrist and a social worker from the Drug Dependency Clinic, and the AIDS Education co-ordinator, amongst others. It was clear from this experience that, in order to gain the confidence of the women, entirely different methods were needed to reach this group.

In September 1987, I was asked by the Regional Drugs and AIDS co-ordinator of the Mersey Regional Health Authority (MRHA) to assist in a small exploratory survey of certain aspects of the sex industry in Merseyside. This request was initially rather intimidating. However, preliminary discussions indicated that there was professional support for the proposed venture from workers at the syringe exchange scheme, the genito-urinary medicine clinic, and welfare agencies. Accordingly, a pilot initiative was launched. It was thought that an informal 'outreach' approach would reach deeper into the hidden sector than conventional health or social work approaches. Outreach, as the name suggests, involves initiating friendly contacts with the target group on their terms, on the streets or other places where they meet (Matthews, 1989).

The main purpose of the project was to assess the knowledge and attitudes of female sex workers in relation to HIV/AIDS and other STD infections, and to design strategies for education and intervention into some of the more high-risk activities in which they might be involved. Field work was undertaken immediately and contact established with the women involved. Although the women were understandably very suspicious at first, trust was established fairly quickly by befriending and demonstrating positive unconditional regard with respect to the women's activities. It was recognized from the outset that, if credibility was to be achieved amongst this group, a non-judgmental approach had to be adopted. To make radical changes to their lives the women needed to feel worthwhile and empowered. Starting from the perspective that what one does is 'bad', or that one's entire life is pathological, would be doomed to failure (Springer, 1991).

As initial contacts developed, a clearer picture emerged of the size and nature of the prostitution scene in Liverpool. Although much of the prostitution scene in the city is difficult to explore (involving call girls, massage parlours, escort agencies, etc), it was possible to identify certain areas where high-profile, street work takes place.

The scene

While an unknown number of women worked from nightclubs, hotels and saunas in the city centre, a sizable and very visible group worked 'the Block', a residential area on the southern periphery of the city centre. This area bears many of the characteristics of what ecological theorists termed a 'zone of transition', low cost, often run-down housing with a diverse group of residents that includes students and a high proportion of Liverpool's indigenous black population, to young urban professionals engaging in the gentrification of Georgian and Edwardian town-houses (McDermott et al., 1988). According to many elderly residents, this area has been operated by prostitutes since the 1950s.

A hard core of fifty to sixty women regularly worked this area, supplemented by a periphal, transient population who work as fortunes dictate. In the main, they would be in their late teens and early twenties, of low socioeconomic background and with a range of personal, social and behavioural problems. It appeared that levels of alcohol and illicit drug use were much higher amongst this group than could be expected of other women their age, which is not surprising given the kind of lifestyle they were involved in. The women worked street corners, with most of the clients picking them up in cars. However, during the frequent police purges on prostitution in the area, the women had to keep 'on the move' to avoid arrest. Although the women will always try to work in pairs, which provides both company and protection, this is not always possible, leaving them vulnerable to physical attack, abuse and robbery.

The business conducted by the women operating the dockland area in the north end of the city differs considerably from that on the Block. Here, a hard core of thirty to forty women regularly worked the area, but this would vary depending on how busy the docks were. These women were generally older and longer established than those who work the Block, and clients were contacted in clubs and bars around the dock locality. However, drug use on Merseyside has affected the sex industry considerably and over the past few years a younger group of women had begun to operate in this area also. Although Liverpool as a port has declined over the past twenty years, there is still regular trade with West Africa, the Far East, South and North America. These women typically spend the evening drinking and dancing with the same client, before accompanying him back to the ship for the rest of the night.

The survey

Apart from gathering anecdotal information which only gave a very generalized picture of the scene, it soon became apparent that some hard evidence was required to support and direct any future initiatives. To this end, a simple anonymous questionnaire was designed by a researcher from Liverpool University. The survey was carried out during a three month period of September to November 1987, with 34 questionnaires being completed by prostitute women whose ages ranged from sixteen to thirty-nine. The results of the survey indicated that illicit drug use among the women was high with 69 per cent reporting using illicit drugs, with the majority citing heroin as their drug of choice. More than half the sample did not know where to find an agency dealing with drug problems and they perceived other health care services as judgmental and were, therefore, unwilling to use them. A large percentage of the women had been in care themselves as children, and many of their own children were also in the care of the local authority. Despite the insistence of many women that they almost always used condoms while 'doing business', the majority also had sexual partners outside work. Almost all stated that they never used a condom for sex with their husbands or other lovers (McDermott, 1988).

As a result of this exercise a number of objectives were defined, both short and long-term. The most obvious course of action was to make condoms and educational materials readily available and to encourage women who needed immediate help to attend appropriate services. It was also felt that, in the long term, a specific health response was needed aimed at providing a more substantial service to this group, who were traditionally apprehensive of interference from health and social agencies.

The project quickly developed into a comprehensive service for the women and provided the first point of contact into services, such as the Drug Dependency Clinics, GUM Clinics and so on. One important priority of this work was contacting those women who were pregnant and using drugs and accessing them into services. Many were reluctant to disclose their pregnancies, for fear of judgmental attitudes or losing their children to social services care. However, it was felt important that these women should be encouraged to take up the vital health care needed, for both themselves and their unborn child.

Meeting Irene

My first encounter with a pregnant woman was on a cold and rainy Monday night in 1987. I had not been working on the project very long when I met Irene, a small, blonde woman in her early twenties. She was standing with a group of women around a telephone box, which was a regular 'pitch' for many of the women who worked the area. She was heavily pregnant and working to buy heroin for herself and her partner. As we stood and talked in the rain, she began to cry and told me how she had already had three children taken into care. She felt no one wanted to help her because she was a drug user and a prostitute. Before I left her she said to me, 'There must be a better life than this'. I was to learn some months later that Irene's baby was placed in the care of the local authority shortly after being born. This left me feeling very sad and frustrated. My own short experience of working with the women had shown me how marginalized they were in society. I felt that more could be done to support women like Irene and there was a definite need for development in service provision in this area of the work.

Irene became a regular contact of mine as she drifted in and out of prostitution, often spending short periods in jail. One night, about two years later, Irene told me she was expecting again. Although she was about five months pregnant, she had not yet seen a doctor or received any antenatal care. After some encouragement, and reassuring her every effort would be made to help her keep the baby, she agreed to be referred into the local Drug Dependency Clinic and was prescribed a maintenance course of methadone.

At this time, the clinic had begun to prioritize pregnant women, recognizing the need for this special group to be in touch with services and also reducing the risks of HIV infection. A pregnant drug user would be taken into treatment straight away, avoiding the long waiting list the clinic had had to impose. The social worker, and other staff members at the clinic, were able to provide practical support for Irene following the birth of her baby. By clinic staff advocating on her behalf, Social Services recognized that not only did the baby need care, but Irene did too. Fortunately, a foster family was available who was willing to take them both. When the baby was born, she went to live with the family who were not only able to offer support and monitor her progress, but also taught her valuable parenting skills. This enabled Irene, for the first time, to care for her child. After a short period with the foster family, and a lot of hard work from Irene, she was able to move into a home of her own.

Receiving a regular daily prescription of methadone, Irene no longer had to work the streets for drug money and was able to rebuild her life. To my knowledge, Irene still cares for her child and has remained fairly stable. However, without that first contact, Irene may not have found a 'better life'. There were many more women who were referred into the Drug Dependency Clinic during my time with the project. This work contributed to an increase in the numbers of women using the service of Liverpool Drug Dependency Clinic by over 30 per cent (Ruben, 1990).

However, entering into treatment did not always prevent the women from working, as a prescription of methadone did not always stop them from continuing to prostitute themselves. If a drug injector was prescribed methadone linctus, which is taken orally, they would still continue to buy heroin to inject. Also, some women would find being 'scripted' freed up money to buy other drugs, such as crack. It must be remembered that treating an addiction to, say, heroin, does not negate the desire to get high on other drugs. They still drank, they still smoked cigarettes, and the use of a range of drugs is a normal part of everyday life for many of the women. Consequently, the script would become a 'flexible friend' to many, using it in exchange for other drugs or money.

This also applied to those women who were working while pregnant. Many women would continue to work right up to the last minute before the birth. Some would even reappear on the streets only a few days after giving birth. As one women put it, 'I still need money, I can't keep borrowing all the time and the social [welfare benefits] is just not enough to live on. I know I've got my medicine [methadone], but where's the money coming from for all the things I need for the baby?'

Changing drug use patterns

In the latter part of 1988 there was a dramatic change in the drug-using behaviour of many of the women I encountered. A fall in purity and availability of street heroin led to many users switching from smoking to injecting, adding further importance to the use of clean equipment, condoms, and knowledge of HIV transmission. Furthermore, the availability and rapid uptake of crack changed not only their drug use, but also their work practices. Smoking cocaine produces an immediate, intense high that can lead to extremely compulsive and obsessional behaviour. Consequently, many of the women began working longer hours and engaged in more high-risk sexual activity to get the money to buy crack. A major concern was women who used crack during pregnancy, because of the damaging effect the drug could have on the fetus. Cocaine use during pregnancy has been associated with increased rates of placental abruption and still births, in utero strokes have also been reported in some of the literature available from America (Kaiser,1990).

The women who used crack during their pregnancies would report the baby 'stiffening up' in the womb when they smoked a rock. One woman, who was expecting her second child and had used crack for several years, told me, 'The baby definitely feels it when I have a rock - and I can tell it doesn't like it'. All the women who smoked crack during their pregnancies felt guilty about their drug use, but appeared to be unable to control it. 'I know I shouldn't be doing it [crack] but it's hard, it's so hard'.

To further complicate matters, crack users often self-medicate with depressants, typically heroin or temazepam (a benzodiazepine), to cushion the extremely unpleasant come down. As the pleasurable effects of crack last only a few minutes the user is left wanting more of the drug or needs to arrest the unpleasant after-effects such as paranoia and anxiety. One woman explained to me, 'I need a hit [of heroin] when I've had a rock. You just feel so fast, everything is racing, you need the brown [heroin] to feel normal again. It's mad'. Another commented, 'When you're wired, you just want it to stop. It's too fast, you can't think straight. A hit brings you right down'. Some of the women also injected temazepam, which led to serious complications such as deep vein thrombosis and abscesses. The consequence of this form of abuse caused one woman to lose her leg shortly after my leaving the project. Poly-drug use at this level led many of the women, whose primary drug was crack, to become dependent on heroin.

The babies born to mothers addicted to crack tended to be smaller and were sometimes premature, but did not exhibit the severe problems associated with the American 'crack-babies' we'd read about in the papers. This may have been due to lower levels of use, easier access to health services, or less deprived conditions. In America cocaine is far cheaper than in Britain, a vial of crack can be bought for only a few dollars. Cocaine still remains relatively expensive in this country, although users report that prices are falling and quality increasing. However, should levels of cocaine use continue to rise in this country, a different picture may start to emerge regarding cocaine-exposed newborn.

Although most of this work took place on the streets, it was also important to gain access to places like 'shooting galleries' and 'crack houses', where drug users would gather to inject heroin or smoke cocaine. Work in this environment was extremely important, as injection practices could be observed, on the spot advice given and clean injecting equipment provided. This also allowed me valuable insight into drug using behaviours and trends, thus enabling the information to be used for further development of drug and HIV services. Although I felt privileged to be allowed into this inner sanctum of drug use, work in this setting is demanding and very stressful and it is easy to feel isolated. To colleagues, particularly managers, this is a totally alien world which they have difficulty understanding. By its absence I learned the value of supervision and support.

Despite what must seem a depressing and disheartening job, working on the project was both enjoyable and rewarding. Practical interventions with the women not only prevented the spread of HIV infection, but also saved many lives. Dina was an example of this. Dina was a small, black woman in her middle twenties and had turned to prostitution to finance her heroin and crack use. Her drug use began to escalate when her children were taken into the care of the local authority, and she began to inject temazepam into her groin. One night, in August 89, I saw Dina limping down the road, her leg was very swollen and I suspected she had a Deep Vein Thrombosis. I insisted that she go to hospital, but Dina argued that she had to continue working. After much persuasion she finally agreed to go to the hospital, where she was admitted with a DVT in her leg. The doctor told her that had her condition been left another day, she would have at least lost her leg - if not her life. During Dina's stay in hospital, she talked about coming off drugs, so I arranged for her to go straight to a detox unit following her discharge from hospital. She then went on to a residential rehabilitation programme away from Merseyside, which she successfully completed. Recently, Dina and I spoke for the first time in four years. She now works at the rehab and is helping others with their drug problems. For Dina, the help, encouragement and understanding that was on offer made a big difference to her life. She told me, 'Having someone who was there all the time, who understood and didn't judge me, made all the difference. But most of all, having someone who cared. I would not have done this on my own, not without the support I got, I probably would be dead now'.

My work taught me that these are invisible women, either ignored, pitied, or whispered about, but for most part they are unknown to us, hidden from our sight, suffering silently and profoundly. When the light finally shone upon this dark side of society's primitive and cruel treatment, I saw that these women were our mothers, our sisters, our daughters.

This chapter is dedicated to the memory of Linda Donaldson, who was murdered in October 1988.

About the author
Lyn Matthews is a Drugs Counsellor at the Merseyside Drugs Council in Southport and has assisted in the development of services for young, recreational drug users. More recently, she initiated and assisted in the development of services for pregnant substance misusers in the Southport and Formby Health Districts. Until April 1992 she was an outreach worker with Liverpool Health Authority.

CHAPTER TEN

Drugs Counselling and the Pregnant Addict

MERSEYSIDE DRUGS COUNCIL

Social stigmatization

In much of our society the regular taking of illegal drugs is still considered a taboo. It is equated with weakness of character, illness and death. Users are at best judged as pathetic and at worst as evil and destructive. Practices such as injecting drugs are viewed as a threat to establishment values, they are vilified by the media and result in the marginalization of those that indulge in them.

The effect of this stigmatization can often push an individual further into the drug sub-culture widening the gap between themselves and the 'establishment' world. Thus an addict will find him/herself on the edge of criminality by the nature of his/her addiction. With a growing tolerance to a relatively expensive commodity, few means to support it and others at hand to lead the way it is no small wonder that many will become firmly enmeshed in a criminal lifestyle and further into the marginalization from mainstream society.

When a drug-using woman becomes pregnant and, for health, social and maybe economic reasons, requires the services that are available for all women, she may avoid or decline them. Fear can be a major factor, not simply for herself or the child, but as a result of stigmatization. This is a fear of being judged negatively, as a drug user, as a woman and as a mother.

For many women, addicted to drugs the arrival of a baby can prove to be a turning point in their lives. It can be a focus for a new strength and acceptance of unique responsibilities. As such it can mean either a passage back to mainstream living or another event in which they fail and fall further behind.

Family support

Many women expecting their first child can expect a great deal of support from parents and extended family. This is more so in the situation where the woman lacks the support of a partner.

In the case of a drug-using woman family relationships have often suffered considerable breakdown. The partner is often either absent of suffering from the effects of drug abuse himself. Pregnancy can sometimes have the effect of a rallying round 'for the baby's sake', however mistrust, acrimony and bitterness make the situation fragile. If there can be some intervention such as a family support group or counselling, fragile relationships can sometimes be strengthened.

Housing and housekeeping

A large proportion of chronic drug users will find themselves in accommodation unsuitable for the raising of young children. Inadequate housing problems are compounded when the user has learnt few coping skills such as preparing meals, shopping or hygiene. Coping with a budget is a problem when one is used to having to finance an addiction to heroin or crack. If the user is making an effort to stay off street drugs, a move away from their known environment is often the only realistic way of sustaining this.

Again the user may not have the skills or the stamina to take their case to the relevant agencies and push for help. Housing agency staff are often mistrustful if they are aware of a drugs problem and there is a feeling that they could be discriminated against if they disclose their status. If this situation is not addressed the user may attempt to make the best of unsuitable conditions and consequently set themselves up to fail. A common understanding of drug-related issues is needed by housing agencies and sensitivity is required to help advocate and support the user to establish herself.

Treatment and health: service provision issues

Ongoing involvement with a drugs agency can be a crucial factor if the mother is to cope successfully with a pregnancy and the new child. Methadone treatment can be a way of stabilizing someone's heroin addiction. By providing a substitute it affords the opportunity to obtain a free, clean supply of drugs and move further away from the learnt lifestyle involved with the blackmarket merry-go-round. Once the user has stabilized their drug intake there is the opportunity to make a decision regarding moderation of intake or even complete detoxification under medical supervision. Many pregnant drug users have used the extra motivation of an expectant child to make a serious and sustained effort to beat their addiction, and some do succeed.

There are other health complications or risks associated with drug misuse that some users will be prone to. Hepatitis is spreading amongst drug users and can be transmitted far easier than the more publicized HIV virus. Vaccination or preventative measures can be readily undertaken when the user is in contact with health agencies. Persistent poor injecting practice can have a debilitating effect on the body and can make it prone to serious infections such as septicaemia. Many users are seriously undernourished by an inadequate diet lacking in vitamins and vital minerals.

A large proportion of women addicted to heroin will experience a cessation of menstruation. Some believe that because of this they cannot get pregnant. This can lead the user to forgo contraception and be unaware of the early signs of pregnancy. These reasons, as well as the fear of authority, being judged as a bad person, or avoidance of facing up to a difficult reality, can mean that many women present to pre-natal or maternity services late into confinement.

It is difficult to offer someone support when they cannot hear you. The first priority when working with drug users is to reach them and inform them that help is at hand. So services within communities and outreach work are vital.

As mentioned above, the time factor is important when working with pregnant drug users. A system of priority status can ensure that valuable time is not wasted and needs can be assessed almost immediately.

Harm reduction is a key phrase in today's service provision. Abstinence is not always a realistic option for users; we must continue to work with those that choose to remain taking drugs. Access to clean injecting equipment and advice on safer injecting can improve the general health of users and reduce the spread of transmittable disease. Free contraception and family planning services can reduce the risk of unwanted pregnancies and sexually transmitted disease.

Merseyside Drugs Council – Liverpool Counselling Service

This agency has a long history of offering counselling to those whose lives are affected by drugs. These can be illegal drug users or prescribed drug users, as well as their parents and families.

The Liverpool Counselling Service offers ongoing support and counselling as well as a referral service to those in need of help from other agencies. Clients usually present in one of two ways; via the drop-in service where they can see the duty counsellor, or by referral from other agencies such as GPs, the probation service or prison.

The agency employs qualified counsellors who have experience of working with drug users. In addition to this one counsellor specializes in working with the families of drug users and supports them one-to-one or in support groups. Access to prescribing is made through the GP Liaison Scheme where users can be helped to find a GP and their progress is monitored through the counselling service. This can be a boon to doctors who, often overstretched themselves, have traditionally found drug users a difficult group to work with effectively.

The agency has established links with local prisons and has found there is a great demand in prisons for effective harm reduction education and the provision of a pathway into services for those who need it when they return to the community.

In addition, those motivated to completely change their lifestyle and totally abstain from drugs may wish to enter a residential rehabilitation programme. This involves assessing clients' suitability for these programmes on behalf of social services, who will provide funds for them to enter one if necessary.

When working with vulnerable clients, who may be disclosing material they have never shared before, issues such as confidentiality and boundaries need to be clearly understood by all parties. As well as the expected qualities of the counsellor such as empathy and sensitivity, a framework for helping can be used. This allows the client to understand and review change in a step-by-step approach. It is not simply a case of listening, it is a challenging approach that recognizes the client's ability to understand their own feelings and tackle important issues, and their readiness to do so.

This framework is probably best illustrated by use of a real case history. No case is ever truly typical; this story however is presented in a form that hopefully demonstrates some of the rationale behind this type of approach. The name and some details have been changed to protect the anonymity of the client.

Anita

In common with many more heroin users today, Anita had had some contact with drugs services. When she progressed on to injecting the drug she had been introduced to the syringe exchange service where she had been accepted without question or fuss. She had suffered some bruising to her arm and a nurse at the syringe exchange had noticed this and offered some advice on safer injecting.

Anita felt accepted not just as a user but as a person in her own right. By not being pressed into others' values and/or persuasions to 'do something' about her drug use, Anita felt comfortable coming into these agencies She felt they accepted her drug use as part of her choices and were not shocked by it. Hopefully any concern she may expect then would be for her as a person, not out of negative judgement of her practices.

The crisis stage

When Anita discovered she was pregnant she was horrified and immediately in distress. She had no plans to start a family and her partner had recently been sent to prison for drug-related offences. She was currently living with two other women users, one of whom was a sex worker.

She asked to speak to a counsellor and, recognizing her crisis situation, she was seen immediately. She had a whole series of dilemmas that appeared to be insoluble and these presented themselves in the initial session as a torrent of questions to herself.

- Did she want a baby?
- Could she cope?
- Should she have this baby or should she consider an abortion?
- Should she stop using heroin – was it damaging the fetus?
- How would the father/family react?

Each issue raised feelings of guilt and despair and with it a craving to use yet more heroin in an attempt to block these feelings.

Most counselling relationships begin in crisis; it is a recognizable stage during which people think, feel and consequently act differently than normal. Everyday routines can become stressful and difficult, the prospect of change is frightening. It is important that the counsellor recognizes this stage and does not attempt to give advice. Decisions made at this time can be seriously regretted later. Careful listening, warmth and empathy are all that is needed before the dilemmas can begin to be reflected on the process of planning begun.

The exploration stage

As the next couple of sessions progressed Anita began to accept her situation and was better prepared to look rationally at her dilemmas. She had yet to make any decision but was readily exploring options. She talked through the different scenarios and tried to imagine how she may feel about them. She looked at her support network and how she could add to this to help her cope. We discussed the option surrounding detoxification and how, when, and if this was likely to be achieved. This involved Anita taking a truly honest review of her drug use which proved to be a breakthrough in itself. We discussed the pros and cons of being prescribed the heroin substitute methadone and its likely effects on both her and the unborn child. She began to talk about her relationship and fears for their future together.

As the crisis subsides, if the client feels comfortable with the counsellor, she is likely to want to explore all aspects of the problem, sometimes over and over again. It is extremely important that the counsellor is thoroughly knowledgeable and up-to-date on the issues surrounding drug use and pregnancy, but does not give advice, impose values or be judgmental. The client should feel that she arrived at her own decisions for she alone will have to live with them.

The result of this could then be that the client later acknowledges she has taken control of her own life and has not been dependant on others. This can have a beneficial effect on self-esteem and confidence.

Decision-making and action

Shortly after this stage Anita made the decision that she wanted to have the baby. Part of the reason was that she felt she needed to tackle her drug use and the baby would give her life some direction and purpose. She still felt very unsure about her relationship with the father but decided to inform him anyway. She was still routinely using heroin and did not want to risk miscarriage by the added strain of immediate detoxification. In view of this she decided to opt for a methadone course aiming to reduce the dosage through the later terms of pregnancy. At this point a referral was made to the Drug Dependency Clinic where she would be seen as a priority and, from there, access to the community midwife with special responsibility for drug users would be established.

Once decisions are made the situation tends to become more real and we can begin to learn to cope with it. We can then prepare to take any actions that are required. This is often the time when we feel better and more energized. Using a drug such as heroin can provide an escape from thinking and feeling about problems and dilemmas and therefore decisions, though readily made by users, will often fail because they are unrealistic. The counselling sessions enabled Anita to examine her thoughts and feelings in open forum and as trust developed she was challenged more often and found it hard to avoid the issues.

Postscript

Life for Anita following her involvement with this agency was hardly straightforward. She managed to come off and stay off drugs during her pregnancy. She had a healthy boy and established a comfortable home with support from her family. When her partner returned from prison he moved in with her and they both relapsed. However, before their situation got completely out of control they contacted the agency and went back onto methadone treatment. They still use heroin occasionally out in general lead a stable life with plenty of love and care for the child. Anita would like to be completely drug free but recognizes her partner is weaker than she and when he uses she gives in. Despite this they have a generally happy relationship and would like another child.

In writing these words we are aware that the drug users we have experience of are usually getting some sort of help and treatment and therefore may not be wholly representative of those presenting to maternity services. It is difficult not to be judgmental if you discover a woman in the early stages of labour wanting to go to the toilet for a 'hit' of heroin. Or when a social worker tells you of a client who arrives at a case conference called about her children stoned and falling asleep.

Both these situations have happened with clients of ours and it is these stories that stick in the mind and are passed around. We were flabbergasted on hearing them as both clients had been very stable for a considerable time. It is only by understanding the user's perception of authority and their fear of being judged and controlled that we could understand why a heroin addict craves and uses their drug in these situations to excess.

By making an extra effort to show compassion and empathy to drug users we can be rewarded with profitable relationships that achieve genuine change. Non-judgmentality in care is the key to achieving this.

About the authors

The Merseyside Drugs Council has operated a counselling service in the heart of Liverpool since the mid-1960s. The agency attempts to address the changing needs and problems created through substance misuse. Experienced counsellors work with both users and family members, helping them develop strategies to overcome the worst effects of addiction.

A priority is to access drug users into primary care and establish contact with other helping agencies. In turn a referral for counselling and support can be made from any individual or organization.

Conclusion

CATHERINE SINEY

Although this book has tried to cover many issues, there are steps that need to be taken to move towards a better service for those vulnerable women and their children.

Education in schools, using project workers, is essential if children are to grow up aware of the problems surrounding drug use. Parents should be educated too.

Accessible and sympathetic support services, both statutory and voluntary, should educate and support in the areas of drugs, contraception and prostitution, as well as health, housing and benefits.

Education and support for student midwives, midwives, midwife teachers, medical staff and social workers must be ongoing. Attitudes are always difficult to change but it helps if people can recognize that they may have an attitude!

There needs to be sharing of research and experience within a combined forum for all professionals acknowledging expertise, experience and commitment to care.

References and Bibliography

Introduction

Advisory Council on the Misuse of Drugs (1993). *AIDS and Drug Misuse Update*. London: HMSO.

Boyd, K. (1990). 'Institute of Medical Ethics: working party report. HIV infection: the ethics of anonymized testing and of testing pregnant women', *Journal of Medical Ethics*, Vol. 16, pp.173–78.

Connaughton, J.F., Reeser, D.S. (1977). 'Management of the pregnant opiate addict: success with a comprehensive approach', *American Journal of Obstetrics and Gynaecology*, Vol. 129 (678), pp.7–8.

Department of Health (1992). 'Department of Health guidance: additional sites for HIV antibody testing; offering voluntary named HIV antibody testing to women receiving antenatal care; partner notification for HIV infection'. PL/CO(92)5.

Institute for the Study of Drug Dependence (1992). *Drugs, Pregnancy and Childcare: a Guide for Professionals*. London.

Kline, J., Stein, Z., Hutzler, M. (1987). 'Cigarettes, alcohol and marijuana: varying associations with birthweight', *International Journal of Epidemiology*, Vol. 16, pp.44–51.

Morrison, C., Siney, C. (1995). 'Maternity services for drug misusers in England and Wales: a national survey', *Health Trends*, Vol. 27, No.1.

Parker, H., Bakx, K., Newcombe, R. (1986). 'Drug misuse in Wirral: a study of eighteen hundred problem drug users known to official agencies'. The First Report of the Wirral Misuse of Drugs Project, University of Liverpool.

Pearson, G. (1987). 'Social deprivation, unemployment and patterns of heroin use'. In: Dorn, N., South, N (Eds). *A Land Fit for Heroin? Drug Policies, Prevention and Practice*. London: Macmillan.

Pearson, G. (1991). 'Drug-control policies in Britain'. In: Tonry, M. *Crime and Justice*. Chicago: University of Chicago Press.

Rooney, C. (Ed.) (1992). *Antenatal Care and Maternal Health: How Effective is it? A Review of the Evidence*. Geneva: WHO.

Siney, C., Kidd, M., Walkinshaw, S., Morrison, C., Manasse, P. (1995). 'Opiate dependency in pregnancy', *British Journal of Midwifery*, February, Vol. 3, No. 2, pp.69–73.

Social Services Inspectorate (1991). 'Community based services for people who misuse drugs: a study in North Western Region'. London: Department of Health.

Standing Conference on Drug Abuse (SCODA), (1989). 'Drug using parents and their children: the second report of the National Local Authority Forum on Drug Abuse in conjunction with SCODA'. London: Association of Metropolitan Authorities.

Tanne, H.J. (1991). 'Jail for pregnant cocaine users in the United States', *British Medical Journal*, Vol. 303, No. 6807, p.873.

Tanne, H.J. (1992). 'Forcing treatment on pregnant women', *British Medical Journal*, Vol. 305, No. 6845, pp.76–77.

UKCC (1989). 'Anonymous testing for the prevalence of human imunodeficiency virus (HIV)'. PC/98/01.

UKCC (1992). Registrar's letter. 24/1992.

UKCC (1993). Registrar's letter. 12/1993.

Chapter One

Dawe, S., Gerada, C., Strang, J. (1992). 'Establishment of a liaison service for pregnant opiate dependent women', *British Journal of Addiction*, Vol. 87, No. 6 June, pp.867–71.

Dixon, A. (1987). 'The pregnant addict', *Druglink*, July/August, pp.6–8.

Fraser, A.C. (1983). 'The pregnant drug addict', *Maternal and Child Health*, November, pp.461–63.

Fraser, A.C., Cavanagh, S. (1991). 'Pregnancy and drug addiction – long term consequences', *Journal of Royal Society of Medicine*, Vol. 84, September, pp.530–32.

Harper, R.G., Solish, G.I., Purow, H.M., Sang, E., Panepinto, W.C. (1974). 'The effect of a methadone treatment programme upon heroin addicts and their newborn infants', *Paediatrics*, Vol, 54, No. 3 September, pp.300–305.

Hepburn, M. (1993). 'Drug use in pregnancy', *British Journal of Hospital Medicine*, Vol. 49, No. 1, pp.51–55.

Strang, J., Moran, C. (1985). 'The pregnant drug addict'. Manchester (unpublished).

Chapter Two

Ashton, H., Golding, J.F. (1989). 'Tranquilizers: prevalence, predictors and possible consequences. Data from a large UK survey', *British Journal of Addiction*, Vol. 84, pp.541–46.

Martin, C.A., Marin, W.R. (1980). 'Opiate Dependence in Women.' In: Kalant, O.J. (Ed.) *Alcohol and Drug Problems in Women*. New York: Plenum.

Medical Working Group on Drug Dependence (1992). 'Guidelines of good clinical practices for the treatment of drug misuse'. London: DHSS.

Rosenbaum, M. (1981). *Women on Heroin*. New Jersey: Rutgers University Press.

Chapter Three

Advisory Council on the Misuse of Drugs (1988). *AIDS and Drug Misuse, Part 1.* London: HMSO.

Banks, A., Waller, T.A.N. (Eds). (1988). *Drug Misuse: A Practical Handbook for GPs.* Oxford: Blackwell Scientific Publication.

Blenheim Project (1990). *Changing Gear: A Book for Women who Use Drugs Illegally.* London: The Blenheim Project/Mental Health Foundation.

El-Palil, A., Bhatacharyya, M. (1994). 'Widespread cutaneous atrophic lesions - signs of an ex-drug user', *British Journal of Sexual Medicine,* Vol. 21 (July.August), pp.35–36.

Hepburn, M. (1992). 'Socially Related Disorders: Drug Addiction, Maternal Smoking and Alcohol Consumption.' In: Calder, A.A., Dunlop, W. (Eds) *High-Risk Pregnancy.* Oxford: Butterworth-Heinemann

Lart, R., Stimson, G.V. (1990). 'National survey of syringe exchange schemes in England', *British Journal of Addiction,* Vol. 85, pp.1433–44.

Moustoukas, N.M., Nichols, R.L., Smith, J.W., Garey, R.E., Egan, R.R. (1983). 'Contaminated street heroin: relationship to clinical infections', *Archives of Surgery,* Vol. 118, pp.746–49.

O'Hare, P.A., Newcombe, R., Matthews, A., Buning, E.C., Drucker, E. (Eds) (1992). *The Reduction of Drug-Related Harm.* London: Routledge.

Reichman, LB., Felton, C.P., Edsall, J.R. (1979). 'Drug dependence: a possible new risk factor for Tuberculosis disease', *Archives of Internal Medicine,* Vol. 139, pp.337–39.

Rementeria, J.L. (Ed.) (1977). *Drug Abuse in Pregnancy and Neonatal Effects.* Saint Louis: CV Mosby Company.

Scott, R.N., Going, J., Woodburn, K.R., Gilmour, P.G., Reid, D.B., Leiberman, D.P., Maraj, B., Pollock, J.G. (1992). 'Intra-arterial temazepam', *British Medical Journal,* Vol.304, p.1630.

Strang, J. and Farrell, M. (1992). 'Harm minimization for drug users: when second best may be first', *British Medical Journal,* Vol 304, pp.1127–28.

Chapter Four

Acker, D., Sachs, B., Tracey, K., Wise, W. (1983). 'Abruptio placentae associated with cocaine use', *American Journal of Obstetric Gynaecology,* Vol. 146, No. 2, pp.220–1.

Allen, M.H. (1991). 'Detoxification considerations in the medical management of substance abuse in pregnancy', *Bulletin of the New York Academy of Medicine,* Vol. 67, No. 3, pp.270–76.

Armer, T.L., Duff, P. (1991). 'Intraamniotic infection in patients with intact membranes and preterm labour', *Obstetric Gynaecology Survey,* Vol. 46, pp.589–93.

Bingol, N., Fuchs, M., Diaz, V. et al. (1987). 'Tertaogenicity of cocaine in humans', *Journal of Paediatrics,* Vol. 110, pp.93–96.

Blinick, G., Wallach, R.C., Jerez, E., Ackerman, B.D. (1976). 'Drug addicition in pregnancy and the neonate', *American Journal of Obstetric Gynaecology*, Vol. 125, pp.135–42.

Chasnoff, I.J., Burns, K.A., Burns, W.T., Scholl, S.H. (1986). 'Prenatal drug exposure: effects on neonates' and infants' growth and development', *Neurotoxicol-Teratol*, Vol. 9(4), pp.311–13.

Chasnoff, I.J., Burns, W.J., Schnoll, S.H., Burns, K.A. (1985). 'Cocaine use in pregnancy', *New England Journal of Medicine*, Vol. 313, p.666–69.

Chasnoff, I.J., Griffith, D.R., Macgrgor, S. et al. (1989). 'Temporal patterns of cocaine use in pregnancy: perinatal outcome', *JAMA*, Vol. 261, pp.1741–44.

Choksi, S.K., Miller, G., Ronione, A. et al. (1989). 'Cocaine and cardiovascular diseases: the leading edge', *Cardiology*, Vol. 3, pp.1–6.

Chouteau, M., Namerow, P.B., Leppert, P. (1988). 'The effect of cocaine abuse on birth weight and gestational age', *Obstetric Gynaecology*, Vol. 72, pp.351–54.

Church, M.W., Dintcheff, B.A., Gessner, P.K. (1988). 'Dose-dependent consequences of cocaine on pregnancy outcome in the Long-Evans rat', *Neurotoxicology and Teratology*, Vol. 10, pp.51–58.

Doberczak, T.M., Kandall, S.R., Wilets, I. (1991). 'Neonatal opiate abstinence syndrome in term and preterm infants', *Journal of Paediatrics*, Vol. 118, No. 6, pp.933–37.

Ellwood, D.S., Sutherland, P., Kent, C., O'Connor, M. (1987). 'Maternal narcotic addiction: pregnancy outcome in patients managed by a specialised drug dependency antenatal clinic', *Australia and New Zealand Journal of Obstetric Gynaecology*, Vol. 27, pp.92–98.

Fantel, A.G., MacPhail, B.J. (1982). 'The teratogenicity of cocaine', *Teratology*, Vol. 26, pp.17–19.

Finnegan, L., Kaltenbach, K., Weiner, S., Haney, B. (1990). 'Neonatal cocaine exposure: assessment of risk scale', *Paediatr Res*, Vol. 27, No. 10A Abstract.

Finnegan, L.P. (1991). 'Treatment issues for opioid dependant women during the perinatal period', *Journal of Psychoactive Drugs*, Vol. 23, No. 2, pp.191–201.

Finnegan, L.P. (1982). 'Outcome of children born to women dependent on narcotics'. In: Stimmel, B. (Ed.). *The Effects of Maternal Alcohol and Drug Abuse on the Newborn*. New York: Haworth Press.

Frank, D.A., Bauchner, H., Parker, S. et al. (1990). 'Neonatal body proportionality and body composition after in utero exposure to cocaine and marijuana', *Journal of Paediatrics*, Vol. 117, p.622–26.

Fricker, H.S., Segal, S. (1978). 'Narcotic addiction, pregnancy and the newborn', *American Journal of Disabled Children*, Vol. 132, pp.360–66.

Fulroth, R., Phillips, B., Durand, D. (1989). 'Perinatal outcome of infants exposed tococaine and/or heroin in utero', *American Journal of Dis. in Child.*, Vol. 143, pp.905–10.

Gillogley, K.M., Evans, A.T., Hansen, R.L. et al. (1990). 'The perinatal impact of cocaine, amphetamine and opiate use detected by universal intrapartum screening', *American Journal of Obstetric Gynaecology*, Vol. 163, pp.1535–42.

Gregg, J.E.M., Davidson, D.C., Weindling, A.M. (1988). 'Inhaling heroin during pregnancy: effects on the baby', *British Medical Journal*, Vol. 296, p.754.

Harper, R.G., Solish, G., Feingol, E. et al. (1977). 'Maternal ingested methadone, body fluid methadone and neonatal withdrawal syndrome', *American Journal of Obstetric Gynaecology*, Vol. 129, pp.417–24.

Harrison, R. (1986). 'The use of non essential drugs, alcohol and cigarettes during pregnancy', *Irish Medical Journal*, Vol. 79, pp.338 –41.

Hepburn, M. (1992). 'Socially related disorders: Drug addiction, maternal smoking and alcohol consumption.' In: Calder, A.A., Dunlop, W. (Eds). *High Risk Pregnancy*. Oxford: Butterworth-Heinemann.

Hepburn, M., Forrest, C.A. (1988). 'Does infection with HIV affect the outcome of pregnancy?', *British Medical Journal*, Vol. 296, p.934.

Hoyme, H.E., Jones, K.L., Dixon, S.D. et al. (1990). 'Prenatal cocaine exposure and vascular disruption', *Paediatrics*, Vol. 85, pp.743–47.

Kaltenbach, K., Finnegan, L.P. (1987). 'Perinatal and developmental outcome of infants exposed to methadone inutero', *Neurotoxicol-Teratol*, Vol. 9(4), pp.311–13.

Klenka, H.M. (1986). 'Babies born in a district general hospital to mothers taking heroin', *British Medical Journal*, Vol. 293, pp.745–46.

Kline, J., Stein, Z., Hutzler, M. (1987). 'Cigarettes, alcohol and marijuana: varying associations with birthweight', *International Journal of Epidemiology*, Vol. 16, pp.44–51.

Krohn, M.A., Hillier, S.L., Lee, M.L., Rabe, L.K., Eschenbach, D.A. (1991). 'Vaginal bacteroides species are associated with an increased rate of preterm delivery among women in preterm labour', *Journal of Infectious Diseases*, Vol. 164, pp.88–93.

Leif, N.R. (1985). 'The drug user as a parent', *International Journal of Addictions*, Vol. 20, pp.63–97.

Little, B.B., Snell, L.M. (1991). 'Brain growth among fetuses exposed to cocaine in utero: asymmetrical growth retardation', *Obstetric Gynaecology*, Vol. 77, pp.361–64.

Little, B.B., Snell, L.M., Klein, V.R. et al. (1989). 'Cocaine abuse during pregnancy: maternal and fetal implications', *Obstetric Gynaecology*, Vol. 73, pp.157–60.

Macgregor, S., Keith, L., Chasnoff, I., Rosner, M., Chisom, G., Shaw, P., Minogue, J. (1987). 'Cocaine use during pregnancy: adverse perinatal outcome', *American Journal of Obstetric Gynaecology*, Vol. 157, pp.686–90.

Mack, G., Thomas, D., Giles, W., Buchanan, N. (1991). 'Methadone levels and neonatal withdrawal', *Journal of Paediatrics, Childcare and Health*, Vol. 27, No. 2, pp.96–100.

Mahalik, M.P., Gautieri, R.F., Mann, D.E. (1980). 'Teratogenic potential of cocaine hydrocholoride in CF-1 mice', *Journal of Pharmacalogical Sciency*, Vol. 69, pp.703–706.

Mahalik, M.P., Gautieri, R.F., Mann, D.E. (1984). 'Mechanisms of cocaine-induced teratogenesis', *Res Commun Substance Abuse*, Vol. 5, pp.279–302.

McDonald, H.M., O'Loughlin, J.A., Vignewaran, R., McDonald, P.J. (1991). 'Vaginal infection and preterm labour', *British Journal of Obstetric Gynaecology*, Vol. 98, pp.427–35.

McGregor, J.A., French, J.I., Richter, R. et al. (1990). 'Antenatal microbiologic and maternal risk factors associated with prematurity', *American Journal of Obstetric Gynaecology*, Vol. 163, pp.1465–73.

Ministerial Group on the Misuse of Drugs (1988). *Tackling Drug Misuse. A Summary of the Government's Strategy (3rd edition)*. London: Home Office.

Oloffson, M., Buckley, W., Anderson, G.E. and Friis-Hansen, B. (1983). 'Investigation of 89 children born to drug-dependent mothers. II. Follow up 1-10 years after birth', *Acta Paediatrica Scandinavica*, Vol. 72, pp.407-10.

Oppenheimer, E., Stimson, G.V., Thorley, A. (1979). 'Seven year follow up of heroin addicts: abstinence and continued use compared', *British Medical Journal*, Vol. 2, pp.627–30.

Oro, A.S., Dixon, S.P. (1987). 'Perinatal cocaine and methamphetamine exposure: maternal and neonatal correlates', *New England Journal of Medicine*, Vol. 297, pp.528–30.

Ostrea, E.M., Chavez, C.J. (1979). 'Perinatal problems (excluding neonatal withdrawal in maternal drug addiction: a study of 830 cases', *Journal of Paediatrics*, Vol. 94, pp.292–95.

Perlmutter, J. (1974). 'Heroin addiction and pregnancy', *Obstetric Gynaecology Survey*, Vol. 29, pp.439–46.

Pond, S.M., Kreek, M.J., Tong, T.G., Raghoutath, J., Berowitz, N.L. (1985). 'Altered methadone pharmokinetics in methadone maintained pregnant women', *Journal of Pharmacological Experimental Therapy*, Vol. 233, pp.1–6.

Rajegouda, B.K., Kandal, J.R., Falcighia, H. (1978). 'Sudden infant deaths in infants of narcotic-dependent mothers', *Early Human Development*, Vol. 2, pp.219–25.

Riley, D. (1987). 'The management of the pregnant drug addict', *Bulletin of the Royal College of Psychiatrists*, Vol. 11, pp.362–65.

Robins, L.N., Mills, J.L., Krulewitch, C., Allen, A.H. (1993). 'Effects of in utero exposure to street drugs', *American Journal of Public Health*, Vol. 83 (Supplement), pp.6–32.

Rosner, M.A., Keith, L., Chasnoff, I.J. (1982). 'Western University Dependence Programme: the impact of intensive prenatal care on labour and delivery outcomes', *American Journal of Obstetric Gynaecology*, Vol. 144, pp.23–27.

Salafia, C.M., Vogel, C.A., Vintzileos, A.M., Bantham, K.F., Pezzullo, J., Silberman, L. (1991). 'Placental pathological findings in preterm birth', *American Journal of Obstetric Gynaecology*, Vol. 165, pp.934–38.

Schwartz, P., Pattinson, R.C., Deale, J., Carstens, A. (1989). 'Subclinical chorioamnionitic infection in preterm deliveries', *Proceedings of the Eighth Conference in Priorities in Perinatal Care,* Mpekweni, Ceskei, South Africa, pp.42–43.

Silver, H., Wapner, R., Loriz-Vega, M., Finnegan, L.P. (1987). 'Addiction in pregnancy: high risk intrapartum management and outcome', *Journal of Perinatology*, Vol. 7(3), pp.178–84.

Smith, C.G., Deitch, K.V. (1987). 'Cocaine: a maternal, fetal and neonatal risk', *Journal of Paediatric Health Care*, Vol. 1, pp.120–24.

Strauss, M.E., Andresko, M., Styker, J.C., Wardell, J.N., Dunkel, L.D. (1974). 'Methadone maintenance during pregnancy: pregnancy, birth and neonatal characteristics', *American Journal of Obstetric Gynaecology*, Vol. 120, pp.895–900.

Sutton, L.R., Hinterliter, S.A. (1990). 'Diazepam abuse in pregnant women on methadone maintenance: implications for the neonate', *Clin. Paediatr. Phila.*, Vol. 29, No. 2, pp.108–11.

Thornton, L., Clune, M., Maguire, R., Griffin, E., O'Connor, J. (1990). 'Narcotic addiction: the expectant mother and her baby', *Irish Medical Journal*, Vol. 83(4), pp.139–42.

Woods, J.R., Plessinger, M.A. (1990). 'Pregnancy increases cardiovascular toxicity to cocaine', *American Journal of Obstetric Gynaecology*, Vol. 162, ppo.529–33.

Woods, J.R., Plessinger, M.A., Clark, K.E. (1987). 'Effect of cocaine on uterine blood flow and fetal oxygenation', *JAMA*, Vol. 257, pp.957–61.

Zuckerman, B., Frank, D.A., Hingson, R. et al. (1989). 'Effects of maternal marijuana and cocaine on fetal growth', *New England Journal of Medicine*, Vol. 320, pp.762–68.

Chapter Five

Alter, M.J. (1994). 'Transmission of hepatitis C virus – route, dose and titre'. Editorial. *N. Eng. J. Med.*, Vol. 330, noll p.784-86.

Beasley, R.P., Trepo, C., Stevens, C.E., Szmuness, W. (1977). 'The e antigen and vertical transmission of hepatitis B surface antigen'. *Am. J. Epidemiol.*, Vol. 105, p. 94-98.

HMSO (1992) *Immunisation against Infectious Diseases.* London: HMSO.

Moradpour, D. and Wands, J.R. (1995). 'Understanding hepatitis B infection'. Editorial. *N Engl J Med*, Vol. 332, No. 16, pp.1092-93.

Teo, C.G. (1992). 'The virology and serology of hepatitis : an overview'. *CDR Review*, Vol. 2, No. 10, R109-14.

Vajro, P. and Fontanella, A. (1991). 'Breastfeeding and hepatitis B'. *J. Paediatr. Gastroenterol. Nutr.* Vol. 12, No. 1, p.141.

Zanetti, A.R., Tanzi, E., Paccagnini S. et al. (1995). 'Mother to infant transmission of hepatitis C virus'. *Lancet,* Vol. 345, No. 8945, p. 289-91.

Chapter Six

Biggar, R.J.B., Paliwa, S., Minkoff, H., et al. (1989). 'Immunosupression in pregnant women infected with Human immunodeficiency virus'. *Amer. J of Obs. and Gyn.,* Vol. 6, No. 5, pp.1239–44.

Communicable Diseases Report. 21st April 1995, Vol. 5, No. 16.

Connor, E.M., Sperling, R.S., Gelber, R., et al. (1994). 'Reduction of maternal-infant transmission of human immunodeficiency virus type 1 with Zidovudine treatment'. *N. Eng. J. of Med.,* Vol. 331, No. 8, pp.1173–225.

De Vincenzi, I. for the European Study Group on heterosexual transmission of HIV (1994). 'A longitudinal study of Human immunodeficiency virus transmission by heterosexual partners'. *N. Eng. J. of Med.,* Vol. 331, No. 6, pp.341-46.

European Collaborative Study (1993). 'Caesarean section and risk of vertical transmission of HIV-1 infection'. *Lancet,* Vol. 343, No. 8911, pp.1464-67.

HMSO (1992). *Immunisation against Infectious Diseases.* London: HMSO.

Newell, M.L., Dunn, D., Peckham, C.S. (1992). 'Risk factors for mother to child transmission of HIV-1. The European Collaborative Study'. *Lancet,* Vol. 339, No. 8800, pp.1007–12.

Newell, M.L. for the European Collaborative Study (1993). 'Natural history of vertically acquired HIV infection.' *Paediatrics,* Vol. 94, No. 6, pp.815–19.

O'Shaughnessy, M.V. and Schechter, M.T. 'Learning about HIV-2'. *Lancet,* Vol. 344, No. 8934, pp. 1380–81.

Selwyn, P.A., O'Connor, P.G. (1992). 'Diagnosis and treatment of substance users with HIV infection'. *Primary Care,* Vol. 19, No. 1, pp.119–55.

Sherrard, J.S., Bingham, J.S., Owen, T.S. (1993). 'Clinical management of HIV disease in intravenous drug users'. *Int. J of STD and AIDS,* Vol. 4, No. 5, pp.254–60.

Tallon, D.F., Corcoran, D.J.D., O'Dwyer, E.M., Greally, J.F. (1984). 'Circulating lymphocyte subpopulations in pregnancy: a longitudinal study'. *J. of Immunol.* Vol. 132, No. 4, pp.1784–87.

Tovo, P.A., De Martino, M., Gabiano, C. et al. (1992). 'Prognostic factors and survival in children with perinatal HIV-1 infection'. *Lancet,* Vol. 339, No. 8804, pp.1249-53.

Chapter Seven

Donoghoe, M.C. 91992). 'Sex, HIV and the injecting drug user', *British Journal of Addiction*, Vol. 87, pp.405–16.

Hepburn, M. (1994). 'Preventing HIV infection in female injecting drug users', *Maternal and Child Health*, Vol. 19, pp.92–95.

Huws, R. (1989). 'Sexual problems and addiction', *British Journal of Sexual Medicine*, Vol. 16, pp.274–79.

Morrison, C.L., Ruben, S.M., Wakefield, D. (1994). 'Female street prostitution in Liverpool', *AIDS*, Vol. 8, pp.1194–95.

Morrison, C.L., McGee, A., Ruben, S.M. (1995). 'Alcohol and drug misuse in prostitutes', *Addiction*, Vol. 90, pp.292–93.

Morrison, C.L., Ruben, S.M., Beeching, N.J. (1995). 'Female sexual health problems in a drug dependency clinic', *International Journal of STD and AIDS*, Vol. 6, pp.201–203.

Morrison, C.L., Siney, C., Ruben, S.M., Worthington, M. (in press). 'Obstetric liaison in drug dependency', *Addiction Research*.

Morrison, C.L. (1993). 'Women, contraception and HIV', *Drug and Therapeutics Bulletin*, Vol. 31, pp.97–98.

Chapter Eight

Adimora, A.A., Hamilton, H., Holmes, K.K., Sparling, P.F. (1994). *Sexually Transmitted Diseases*. Companion Handbook. Second Edition. USA: McGraw-Hill Inc.

Katz, V.L., Moos, M.K., Cefalo, R.C. et al (1994). 'Group B streptococci: Results of a protocol of antepartum screening and intrapartum treatment.' *Am. J. Obstet. Gynecol.*, Vol. 170, No. 2, pp. 521–26.

McGregor, J.A., French, J.I., Milligan, K. et al (1994). 'Bacterial vaginosis is associated with prematurity and vaginal fluid mucinase and sialidase: Results of a controlled trial of topical clindamycin cream.' *Am. J. Obstet. Gynecol.*, Vol. 170, No. 4, pp.1048–58.

Chapter Nine

Kaiser, M. (1990). 'Cocaine exposed newborns'. *Paedriatric Review*. New Orleans: Children's Hospital.

Matthews, L. (1989). 'Outreach work with female prostitutes in Liverpool'. In Plant, M. (Ed.) *Aids, Drugs and Prostitution*. Tavistock/Routledge.

McDermott, P. et al. (1988). *Prostitutes, Drugs and HIV Infection*. Mersey Regional Health Authority.

Ruben, S. (1990). 'The implications for drug dependency units'. In: Henderson, S. (Ed.) *Women HIV Drugs*. London: ISDD.

Springer, E. (1991). 'Effective AIDS prevention with drug users; the harm reduction model'. In *Counselling Chemically Dependent People With HIV Illness*. Haworth Press.

Further Reading

Adimora, A., Hamilton, H., Holmes, K.K., Sparling, P.F. (1994). *Sexually Transmitted Diseases*. 2nd edition. Companion Handbook. USA: McGraw-Hill.

AIDS (1994) 'A Year in Review'. *Current Science*.

Ashton, J. et al. (1989). *The New Public Health*. Liverpool: Liverpool University Press.

Carmen, A. (1985). *Working Women*. Harper and Row.

Corcoran, G.D., Ridgway, G.L. (1994). 'Antibiotic chemotherapy of bacterial sexually transmitted diseases in adults: a review.' *Int. J. of STD and AIDS*, 5, pp.165–71.

Gleicher, N. (1994). *Principles and Practice of Medical Therapy in Pregnancy*. 2nd edition. Appleton and Large.

Matthews, L. (1993). 'Outreach on the front line'. *Druglink*. ISDD. Vol. 8 Issue 2.

Sande, M.A. and Volberding, P.A. (1994) *The Medical Management of AIDS*. Philadelphia: W.B. Saunders

Sherlock, S. and Dooley, J. *Diseases of the Liver and Biliary System*. Ninth Edition.Oxford: Blackwell Scientific Publications.

APPENDIX ONE

Liverpool Neonatal Drug Withdrawal Chart

LIVERPOOL NEONATAL DRUG WITHDRAWAL CHART

Name: _____ Casenote No:_____ D.O.B: _____Gestation: _____

All infants of drug misusers must have observations started from birth.
Observations made post-feed.
Severe symptoms - please tick (✓) if present.

	Date: Time:								
1. Convulsions									
2. Tremors when undisturbed. Non-stop high pitched cry. Sleeps < 1 hr after good feed. (All must be present to score)									
3. Watery stools or projectile vomiting and requirement of tube feeds									
Signature:									

	Date: Time:								
1. Convulsions									
2. Tremors when undisturbed. Non-stop high pitched cry. Sleeps < 1 hr after good feed. (All must be present to score)									
3. Watery stools or projectile vomiting and requirement of tube feeds									
Signature:									

	Date: Time:								
1. Convulsions									
2. Tremors when undisturbed. Non-stop high pitched cry. Sleeps < 1 hr after good feed. (All must be present to score)									
3. Watery stools projectile vomiting and requirement of tube feeds									
Signature:									

See overleaf for
instructions on treatment.

LIVERPOOL NEONATAL DRUG WITHDRAWAL CHART

INSTRUCTIONS FOR TREATMENT

Minor Symptoms need not be recorded.

(Minor symptoms listed for differentiation purpose - tremors when disturbed, respiration's > 60 per minute, pyrexia of unknown origin, sweating, frequent yawning, sneezing / nasal stuffiness, poor feeding / regurgitation, loose stools). If treatment of the 3 severe symptoms not judged clinically necessary, then reasons must be recorded in casenotes.

Treatment: 0.04 mg / kg morphine sulphate orally. Begin treatment 4 hourly ("treatment level 5"). Then reduce level of treatment every 24 hours if severe symptoms not present as follows:

0.04 mg / kg morphine sulphate 6 hourly ("treatment level 4 ")
0.04 mg / kg morphine sulphate 8 hourly ("treatment level 3")
0.04 mg / kg morphine sulphate 12 hourly ("treatment level 2")
0.04 mg / kg morphine sulphate   daily ("treatment level 1")

If severe symptoms still present do not reduce level.

If severe symptoms persist on 4 hourly morphine ("treatment level 5") discuss with senior paediatrician the possibility of increasing dose of morphine or adding other medication.

Poster

<u>Liverpool Women's Hospital</u>

Are you pregnant or thinking about becoming pregnant?

Are you misusing substances whether prescribed or illicit?

If the answer to this is YES

there is confidential help and information
available from a specialist midwife
who will be able to advise you about
your pregnancy.

Please ring 0151 708 9988

and ask for the specialist midwife or,
leave a message (Ext. 4014, answerphone) and
she will contact you.

Or you can ask at your GPs reception
(or the reception of this department).

APPENDIX THREE

The Liverpool Women's Hospital

Information about the Care of Pregnant Substance Abusers

All substance abusers should be notified to the drug liaison specialist midwife. The specialist midwife is notified routinely by the prescibing agency (or GP) or directly by the records clerks or the midwives/doctors at booking. Some unregistered women may be known only to her.

All known substance abusers are booked under either Mr Walkinshaw or Mr Kidd. The specialist midwife can book direct to each consultant.

Care may be shared with the GP (if they have one and if the consultant thinks this appropriate) or the specialist midwife or both.

Some women may only see the specialist midwife. If the women are booked in drug clinics or 'drop-ins' or at home the specialist midwife will arrange for an ultrasound scan and a hospital appointment. The specialist midwife sees substance abusers at least monthly throughout pregnancy, if they are not attending antenatal services elsewhere.

Registered addicts may receive methadone (opiate substitute) from drug clinics (which clinic depends on postcode), GPs or via probation or the Merseyside Drugs Council (MDC).

The methadone regime advised by the drug prescribing units is stabilisation in the first trimester, reduction (if possible) in the second trimester, by a maximum of 5mg per week, and maintenance in the third trimester. (GPs may not follow this prescribing regime.) Some women do reduce up to the end of the pregnancy, but this should only be tried if they are stable. It is better not to reduce methadone if they are going to increase heroin. Reduction should be encouraged and neonatal withdrawals should be explained, together with the treatment the baby may require.

Advice re. prescribing for unregistered drug users may be obtained during office hours from Dr Clive Morrison – obstetric liaison based at the Maryland Centre, 8 Maryland Street, L1, 0151-709-2231.

The risk from unmonitored or sudden opiate withdrawal either in pregnancy or during labour should be emphasised. (Because opiate withdrawal may make the uterus irritable early or premature labour may be disguised and opiate abusers may not be able to tell the difference; it may precipitate labour.)

All drug abusers are routinely offered a blood test for Hepatitis B and C (please request HBsAg and Anti HBc and Anti HCV on the PHLS virology form). They are not offered HIV testing; if a substance abuser requests HIV testing they should be referred to the relevant drugs agency (information from specialist midwife). There is a unit HIV testing protocol available (info from specialist midwife). Urine may only be tested for drugs if the woman has given permission.

Methadone is given as prescribed during labour together with any analgesia required. It is prescribed as a daily dose at any time that the women are in-patients, they may ask for it any time and may split up their dose during a 24 hour period; (they may not ask for all that they are prescribed.)

The hospital pharmacy have a list of methadone users (regularly updated), the amount of methadone they are prescribed and who prescribes it. (Pharmacy guidelines are available on each ward/dept.) The specialist midwife also tells the pharmacy of non-registered opiate addicts and the approximate amount of opiate, if known.

Withdrawal from opiates in labour may be shown by fetal distress on the CTG monitor, therefore it is helpful to ensure that the woman has an adequate amount of opiate throughout labour, so that the opiate withdrawal induced fetal distress can be excluded from other obstetric emergencies.

Our own research (comparing 103 treated opiate users with controls) has shown that opiate users in labour use 'normal' amounts of analgesia provided that methadone levels are maintained. Unregistered (i.e. untreated) opiate users may require larger amounts of opiates for pain relief in labour, unless methadone is given to stabilise withdrawal in the woman.

Discharge is after 72 hours (this matches the paediatric protocol for infants of substance abusers) because our research has shown that neonatal withdrawal symptoms (from methadone, which has a longer half life than heroin) generally occur (if at all) after 24 hours and if they have not occurred by 72 hours, or if they begin to occur in mild form at that stage, i.e. after 72 hours, there is no problem after discharge. Babies which have severe symptoms are treated as per the paediatric protocol, which is included in the neonatal withdrawal chart. Mothers and babies are kept together and use any bed in the postnatal area; no isolation and no special control of infection procedures are required.

All substance abusers known to the specialist midwife are reviewed regularly by the specialist midwife and the hospital social workers, and the need for formal social service input will be decided by them prior to the birth of the infant.

If any further information is required please contact Catherine Siney – Drug Liaison Specialist Midwife – 0151-708-9988 Ext 4104 or BT Bleep 0893-955118.

OTHER NEW TITLES FROM BOOKS FOR MIDWIVES PRESS

A SHORT HISTORY OF CLINICAL MIDWIFERY
The Development of Ideas in the Professional Management of Childbirth

Philip Rhodes

A Short History of Clinical Midwifery is an illustrated review of the general and historical progress made in clinical midwifery and obstetrics throughout the centuries. It charts the development of the conquest of difficult labour, pain, haemorrhage, infection and eclampsia among many other things and examines how we have arrived at the present situation in the theory and management of childbirth.

Chapters include: The Beginnings: Hellenic times; The Bible; Hellenistic and Roman times; Renaissance; Seventeenth Century: The Handy Operation; The Origin of the Obstetric Forceps; Eighteenth Century: William Smellie; Eighteenth Century: Other Advances; Progress in the Nineteenth Century; Mortality Statistics

Price £17.95   **ISBN 1 898507 22 8**

COMMUNICATING MIDWIFERY
Caroline Flint

Communicating Midwifery is a collection of articles by Caroline Flint, President of the Royal College of Midwives, and one of the profession's most renowned author/practitioners. Caroline's amusing and informative writing traces the development of the midwifery profession over the last twenty years. She has the ability to articulate and make public the issues which have concerned, irritated, excited, frustrated and saddened midwives everywhere - from everyday topics such as uniform to far reaching developments like 'Changing Childbirth'. Her writing is a source of inspiration to all midwives regardless of their place of work and type of practice.

Caroline's articles cover all aspects of midwifery including : Home birth; Teams and caseloads; Clinical issues; Attitudes to childbirth; Legal aspects and Midwifery supervision.

Price £12.95   **ISBN 1 898507 19 8**

SUPER-VISION
Recommendations of the Consensus Conference of Midwifery Supervision

Association of Radical Midwives

The eagerly awaited report of this important conference, during which the delegates formed six discussion groups, each exploring a different aspect of the subject, and putting forward their recommendations for improvements in midwifery supervision. The topics for discussion were selection, preparation and education, communication, the conflicting roles of 'policeman' and 'friend', clinical credibility and accountability.

The conference speakers were drawn from a wide range of midwifery fields - clinical practice, management, supervision, research, education, as well as from other disciplines such as social work and psychotherapy. Each speaker has contributed an essay which expands on the conference themes.

Price £9.95   **ISBN 1 898507 34 1**

WATERBIRTH
Dianne Garland

An up-to-date examination of the use of hydrotherapy in midwifery practice providing guidelines for waterbirth practice in hospital or at home. With the continuing increase in the use of complementary therapies, this book is a timely resource and an invaluable guide for both health care professionals and parents.

Subjects covered include : Midwife accountability; International perspectives on waterbirth, especially USA and Belgium; Setting up a waterbirth facility; Maternal and fetal perspectives; Current research issues; What If ? - Complications and problems; Professional and parental accounts of waterbirths; Early pioneers of waterbirth eg. Odent and Rosenthal; Antenatal and postnatal use of hydrotherapy eg. aquanatal classes.

Includes useful addresses eg. birthing tub companies.

PRICE £10.95   **ISBN 1 898507 33 3**

OTHER TITLES FROM BOOKS FOR MIDWIVES PRESS

TEACHING PHYSICAL SKILL FOR THE CHILDBEARING YEAR	**Brayshaw & Wright**	£10.95
HIV IN PREGNANCY	**Caroline Shepherd**	£ 6.95
ANTENATAL INVESTIGATIONS	**Maureen Boyle**	£ 6.95
UNDERSTANDING OBSTETRIC ULTRASOUND	**Jean Proud**	£10.95
MIRIAD	**NPEU**	£14.95
AQUANATAL EXERCISES	**Gillian Hawksworth**	£ 6.95
HOLDING ON?	**Hazel McHaffie**	£ 9.95
REACTIONS TO MOTHERHOOD	**Jean Ball**	£10.95
SEXUALITY AND MOTHERHOOD	**Irene Walton**	£10.95
LEGAL ASPECTS OF MIDWIFERY	**Bridgit Dimond**	£12.95
MIDWIVES AND 'CHANGING CHILDBIRTH'	**Walton & Hamilton**	£ 9.95

Please order Books for Midwives Press titles from your usual bookseller and encourage them to stock midwifery titles. If you prefer you can order direct from us by sending a cheque, made payable to Books for Midwives Press, to 174a Ashley Road, Freepost WA1836, Hale, Cheshire, WA15 9BR.

All UK orders are sent postage free. For overseas orders please add 25% of total price for postage and packing.

Customers wishing to pay by credit or debit card (Access, Visa, Switch or Delta) can call our hotline on 0161-929-0929.

If you would like to see a copy of our catalogue or to receive information about forthcoming titles, please send us your name, address and telephone number and we will add your name to our mailing list.

Please quote the reference **PDA1** on any orders or correspondence.